The
Silenced
Child

Also by Claudia M. Gold, MD

Keeping Your Child in Mind

THE SILENCED CHILD

From Labels, Medications,
and Quick-Fix Solutions
to Listening, Growth,
and Lifelong Resilience

Claudia M. Gold

A Merloyd Lawrence Book
DA CAPO PRESS
A Member of the Perseus Books Group

Designed by Janelle Fine
Set in 11.5 Goudy Old Style by the Perseus Books Group

Cataloging-in-Publication data for this book is available from the Library of Congress.

First Da Capo Press edition 2016
ISBN: 978-0-7382-1839-7
ISBN: 978-0-7382-1840-3 (e-book)

Published as a Merloyd Lawrence Book by Da Capo Press, A Member of the Perseus Books Group

www.dacapopress.com

The information in this book is true and complete to the best of our knowledge. This book is intended only as an informative guide for those wishing to know more about health issues. In no way is this book intended to replace, countermand, or conflict with the advice given to you by your own physician. The ultimate decision concerning care should be made between you and your doctor. We strongly recommend you follow his or her advice. Information in this book is general and is offered with no guarantees on the part of the authors or Da Capo Press. The authors and publisher disclaim all liability in connection with the use of this book.

The families described in this book are composites of many actual families. All names and identifying details have been changed. Any similarity to actual persons is coincidental.

Da Capo Press books are available at special discounts for bulk purchases in the U.S. by corporations, institutions, and other organizations. For more information, please contact the Special Markets Department at the Perseus Books Group, 2300 Chestnut Street, Suite 200, Philadelphia, PA 19103, or call (800) 810-4145, ext. 5000, or e-mail special.markets@perseusbooks.com.

10 9 8 7 6 5 4 3 2 1

For my father

There is only one cardinal rule. One must always *listen* to the patient.

–*Oliver Sacks in* Migraine
New York Vintage 1999

Contents

Introduction

The Power of Listening

Three-year-old Cara, in a bright polka-dotted dress and slightly uneven pigtails, smiles impishly in to the camera. "You see she's standing on the kitchen table," her proud yet concerned grandmother, Anne, says to me. She shows me the photo and explains that Cara was standing on the table because she "never listens," and runs away when her mother tries to take her picture.

Anne knows that I am a pediatrician and "expert" in behavior problems, so, after showing me the picture, she mentions that her granddaughter might have ADHD (attention-deficit/hyperactivity disorder). "She won't sit in the circle with the other kids for the whole story time. They've started an evaluation."

Anne is my neighbor. Out gardening on the first warm day of spring, she saw me walking my dog and invited me in for tea. As I listen to her story, I nod in shared concern, and she goes on. We've known each other for many years, so the conversation flows easily. "It's hard," she says, "because Mindy (her daughter) just broke up with her boyfriend." "So, she's a single mom," I say. "Yes, and she works late and lets Cara stay up until eleven so she can be with her." After a pause I comment, "So, Cara must be tired in school." Cara's grandmother goes on to explain that Cara is the youngest in her class of mostly four-year-olds. She begins to wonder whether all these things she is telling me might be related to the problems Cara is having in school. Her tone shifts.

Then she reflects, "Actually, Mindy was like that as a child. She took everything in—all the lights and sounds—and could be easily distracted. But after some struggles during those years, she found her way."

During my visit I feel a shift in Anne's thinking. Simply by talking with me, a captive audience with whom she has a long-standing relationship, she goes from describing her granddaughter in terms of a "disorder" and "evaluations" to reflection about Cara, to wondering, "Why is she behaving that way?"

Anne again looks at the giddy expression of her granddaughter, trapped on the kitchen table. She sees the picture, cute as it is, as a kind of sign that things may feel out of control for Cara. She shares with me a concern that perhaps her daughter is too stressed and needs more help from her. Maybe, she says, if Mindy had a bit of time to herself, she could be more patient with Cara. Anne decides to offer her daughter a day of babysitting.

When her grandmother was given the opportunity to wonder about the meaning of that photo, she could understand that Cara's behavior was a way of communicating. Being heard and recognized in this way gave Anne the opportunity to see Cara not as a child with a possible disorder, but instead one who is expressing her needs in the best way she can.

This brief vignette captures the shift from focus on behavior to curiosity about the meaning of behavior, a shift that, as we will see throughout this book, is essential for supporting healthy emotional development. It captures how that shift can occur when we protect space and time for listening to each other.

The thesis of this book is that a culture of advice, quick fixes, parent training, and behavior management, together with a rapidly escalating use of psychiatric labels and medications, may actually interfere in development if parents are not supported in listening to what their child's behavior is communicating.

The evidence for this thesis, and so the backbone of this book, is in the stories themselves, stories (with details changed to protect privacy) that have been told to me by parents and children over the course of twenty-five years practicing pediatrics. Behind every "behavior problem" is a story that gives meaning to that behavior.

The book aims to speak to all who have opportunity to support children like Cara, including family members as well as professionals—pediatricians, social workers, psychiatrists, teachers, childcare workers, and a range of others. It speaks to all those who are in a position to help set any child who hits the inevitable bumps in the road on the journey of growing up, on a path of growth, healing, and resilience.

Our humanity lies in our history, in the stories we tell of our lives, and the meaning we make of our experience. Stories can be found in families of every kind all over the world. Some are heard. Many are not.

Simply Listening

> I would not give a fig for the simplicity this side of complexity, but I would give my life for the simplicity on the other side of complexity.
>
> —*Oliver Wendell Holmes*

The listening described in this book refers to an act that is simple, but on the "other side of complexity." This kind of listening can heal. It can help children develop a healthy brain and mind. True listening comes from a stance of "not knowing," in which we are open to imagining our way into another's feelings, even when they are not our own. Listening requires a willingness to stay present with difficult, intense feelings while at the same time conveying a feeling of safety, offering another person a sense of being held securely. Most important and most challenging, listening requires being mindful of how our own feelings, memories, and experiences are stirred up; to be fully present, we must be able to manage our own reactions.

Listening to a child in this way is known in developmental psychology as *holding a child's mind in mind*, or what I have shortened in my work to *holding a child in mind*. Over forty years of longitudinal research has shown that this kind of listening promotes flexible thinking, well-regulated emotions, social adaptation, and overall mental health.

Similar concepts of listening can be found in Buddhist thought. Thich Nhat Hanh refers to "compassionate listening."

> When communication is cut off, we all suffer. When no one listens to us we become like a bomb ready to explode. Restoring communication is an urgent task. . . . When we listen with our whole being, we can diffuse a lot of bombs. . . . If there is someone capable of sitting calmly and listening with his or her heart for one hour, the other person will feel great relief from his suffering.

Listening to parents helps them listen to their children. Listening to children, in turn, has been shown to modify the way a child responds to stress, and protects against long-term negative effects of stress on the brain and the body. While genetic inheritance plays a role, holding children in a safe, secure caregiving environment affects the way genes are expressed. The field of epigenetics teaches us there is ample opportunity throughout development to change the impact genes have on the brain and on behavior.

We learn to listen by being listened to. As we will see in Chapter 3, our ability to listen in this way, to find our way into another person's experience, begins to develop in our earliest months of life when parents naturally respond to our wordless communication. Our ability to listen is enhanced in a setting of connection and communication. Alternatively, our ability to listen can atrophy in an environment that does not model or value listening.

My career as a pediatrician has spanned the era in which modern biological psychiatry has become mainstream, and with it, we have seen exponential increases in children being diagnosed with psychiatric disorders and prescribed psychiatric drugs. We have seen a massive cultural shift, with such things as ADHD clinics and the fifteen-minute "med-check" becoming the standard of care.

Recent statistics indicate that diagnosis of ADHD has increased 42 percent in eight years, with one third of cases diagnosed before age six. Three-year-old Cara might be on her way to joining that statistic. From 2012 to 2014, the diagnosis of autism rose from 1 in 88 to 1 in 68, a 30 percent increase. A 4,000 percent rise in diagnosis of childhood bipolar disorder was seen from the time it was first identified in 1990 through the early 2000s. These and other diagnoses, such as anxiety disorder, occur in parallel with the rise in prescribing of psychiatric medication to children. Over the past twenty-five years, we have seen a close to 500 percent increase in the number of children prescribed stimulant medication for ADHD.

My interest in an alternative, preventive approach developed out of what I observed in my clinical work as a general and behavioral pediatrician, and is supported by new advances in developmental science showing how the brain grows in relationships. I have been increasingly struck by the contrast between, on the one hand, the powerful transformations that happen in the quiet space of my office when I simply listen to parents, when children feel heard and understood, and on the other, the current practice that invokes behavior management and may reduce a child's experience to a list of symptoms, a label, and a drug.

Both psychoanalysis and Buddhism maintain that it is the presence of mind of another person that is responsible for healing emotional pain. *Being with* and *bearing witness* are other phrases that describe this phenomenon. When we leap to take—or prescribe—a pill we run the risk of skipping this step.

Biological psychiatry is based on a search to identify an illness. This approach proposes that "there is something wrong with you and I will fix it." In his 2015 keynote address to the International Psychoanalytic Association, Christopher Bollas proposed using the term *mental pain* rather than *mental illness*. A Buddhist approach might suggest instead *mental suffering*. An alternative to the illness model seeks to alleviate suffering and to find and support a strong, healthy self.

Listening to Distress

When our children struggle, an urge to fix the problem is a natural response. But psychoanalyst Sally Provence wisely offered a more appropriate stance: "Don't just do something, stand there and pay attention."

When we don't listen, whether as a parent, friend, or professional, most often it is because we are overwhelmed. The part of our brain needed to reflect on how to help may shut down in the face of distress. We want to help, but we feel helpless. We want to "do something." But without listening, these jumps to action may inadvertently close off, or silence, a child's communication. When we pause for a moment of human connection and communication, we discover a path to healing.

In a recent visit to my office, Jennifer, mother of three-month-old George, described such a situation. She and her husband were fighting all the time. He worked long hours and had little left to offer her at the end of the day. She was struggling with feelings of anxiety that had plagued her much of her life, but which had worsened during her pregnancy. Although she felt her milk supply was good, George's pediatrician had suggested she supplement with formula, because at the last visit George had not gained sufficient weight. This ran counter to Jennifer's own intuition, as she observed what she felt to be a robust and healthy baby.

The pediatrician, suspecting a possible connection between poor weight gain and Jennifer's emotional struggles, had referred the pair to me. Jennifer exuded anxiety. She held her body tensely, speaking in clipped, terse sentences while her long hair partially obscured her face. After we spoke for a while, George, who had been sleeping in his carrier, began to fuss. She looked at me uncertainly. "Should I give him the bottle now?" she asked. I responded with a question, asking her what she thought was best for George. After a moment of uncertainty, she said she would nurse him. When I nodded, she brought him to her breast. Over the course of the next forty-five minutes, as she shared more of her story, she saw him through nursing, fussing, burping, and more nursing, until he was quiet and calm, offering me a delighted smile as he sat comfortably on her lap. Jennifer swept her hair from her face and looked lovingly at her baby, her whole body relaxed in pleasure.

As our visit came to an end, Jennifer's overwhelmed feelings reemerged. "What do I do to protect him from the stress, from my anxiety?" We agreed she needed to continue treatment for her anxiety, and she and her husband needed to work to reconcile their differences.

But she answered her own question. She looked at her peaceful, content baby and said, "I want to focus on being with George. He seems to be doing well." "Yes," I replied.

A few weeks later Jennifer came with George and her husband, Eric. Motivated by the growth she saw in George—he was now gaining weight—she wanted her husband to join her in supporting his healthy development. Our first visit had demonstrated to her just how connected George was, and she was able to demonstrate this to Eric. The three exchanged grins of delight as George, so sensitive and attuned to their emotional state, cooed happily while kicking his legs from the blanket on the floor. At his six-month well visit to the pediatrician, George was thriving. Jennifer's anxiety had abated; her mood and spirits were much improved.

Connectedness regulates our physiology and protects against the harmful effects of stress. Charles Darwin, in a work of great observation and insight, though less well known than the *Origin of Species*, addresses the evolution of the capacity to express emotion. He identifies the highly intricate system of facial muscles, and similarly complex systems of muscles modulating tone and rhythm, or prosody, of voice that exist only in humans. These biologically based capacities indicate that emotional engagement is central to our evolutionary success.

Listening to distress in a child takes strength and endurance. "Breathe through it" is a phrase my yoga teacher, Ilana Siegal, uses during the plank position, which similarly calls for both. To me, breathing through plank is a good metaphor for just listening when a child is struggling.

Recently, in a mother-baby group, Susan described the process of making sense of her three-month-old daughter Avery's distress. She told the group that after a few rough months, she had let go of the desperate need to "make her stop crying." Instead, Susan gave herself time and space to listen to what Avery was trying to communicate. After a number of mismatches, Susan recognized that her daughter became calm when she put her down on her back. Avery showed her delight with her mother's discovery by kicking her legs and cooing responsively. "It was a real conversation," Susan said, "even though she doesn't talk." Then she added, "It felt so good."

When my son Eli was young, he would eat only three foods—bagels, pasta with pesto, and chicken fingers. His resistance was powerful—attempts to offer new foods precipitated not only a meltdown, but also actual gagging in the face of certain smells and tastes. This behavior occurred in the context of a similarly intense reaction to fireworks, a county fair, and any other highly stimulating environment. Recognizing that his food refusal had some kind of physical basis, we hung in there and did not force the issue.

Now seventeen years old, he is an accomplished actor and musician. Recently he performed in Shakespeare's *Henry V* as Pistol, who in a famous scene is forced to eat a raw leek. Eli gagged onstage, offering a performance so effective that audience members worried that his reaction was real. But they were soon comforted when the lights dimmed and, alone onstage, he delivered a poignant, passionate soliloquy.

When I think back on those early years and the many things that were difficult for him, I feel as though I was in a sense holding a long plank pose. I mustered all the strength I could, drawing on the support of family members, friends, and my own therapist, to breathe through it and give him time and space to grow into himself. As I will elaborate on throughout the book, this process called for both finding ways to adapt to his particular vulnerabilities, as well as to transform what were challenges as a child into the strengths he now has as a young man.

When I observe Susan's joy in being able to patiently listen to her baby through that difficult moment, similar to the way I held my son through many such moments, I see a theme common to many parents. Our culture of advice and quick fixes creates an illusion, as I often hear from families in my behavioral pediatrics practice, that as parents we need to "do something" before it's "too late." Resisting that urge is far from easy. It requires great strength and a community, one that may consist of fellow parents, family, teachers, friends, and therapists, as supports and guides during times of uncertainty.

Comfort in Being Heard

There is a deep truth to the adage "One is only as happy as one's least happy child." By pointing this out, I am not advocating for placing a child's needs above a parent's, or what is sometimes termed child-centric parenting. Nor am I referring to the unhappiness of missing a party or afterschool activity. Rather, I am referring to the pain that can come with real struggle, such as a hard-to-console infant, a toddler who has multiple meltdowns on family outings, or the school-age child who is repeatedly left out of social events. There are a myriad of painful challenges our children may face on the path to adulthood.

When our children struggle, we feel hurt on many levels. On the most basic level is our close identification with the child who is a part of us. One mother described hearing her infant's relentless crying as akin to "having my fingernails removed." What hurts them hurts us. Then there may be feelings of guilt or shame about being a "bad parent." Sometimes the pain is even deeper, as when a child's behavior provokes memories of a troubled relationship from our own past. In these situations, as parents we may have behaved in ways we are not proud of—yelling at or ignoring a child whose distress is too much to bear.

If we use the Buddhist view of the word *suffering* as being an ordinary human condition, then without exception, every parent whose child is struggling suffers. When we closely identify with our children, their struggling may be experienced as a reflection on us, making it difficult to hear what they are communicating. When as parents we are given space and time to be heard, such suffering can be relieved. Then we can better hear our children.

Many families come to see me in the wake of a frightening diagnosis for their young child. Teachers, doctors, family members, and friends may have mentioned such labels as "ADHD" and "anxiety disorder." Increasing numbers arrive worried about bipolar disorder. When I first sit with parents, with a full hour ahead of us to hear the story, I find that a calm exterior often belies a complex well of pain.

Consider Angela, the mother of four-year-old Michael, whose multiple tantrums filled their days. She was looking for tips to manage his behavior. His pediatrician and teachers had raised the question of ADHD. Angela wondered about anxiety and OCD (obsessive-compulsive disorder). Mealtime was a primary battleground. Because she was so fearful of precipitating a tantrum, she was feeding Michael herself every meal, literally placing the food in his mouth. She recognized that this was wrong, but she could not get out of this pattern of behavior.

At the start of our first visit, when I met with Michael's parents alone, Angela's tone was practical and matter-of-fact. But when I offered time to listen to her whole story, her voice began to tremble as she connected with the grief around her troubled relationship with her son. Michael had been a challenging child from birth, intense and difficult to soothe. Angela had struggled with postpartum depression. She described a fraught relationship with her own mother, who was "cold and distant." She had two much younger sisters for whom she had been made responsible. She used the same word, *resentment*, to describe her feelings about Michael and her sisters. When Michael turned two and began in a developmentally appropriate way to say no, Angela found herself full of rage. She wept as she told me how such typical behaviors as resisting a bath would precipitate an extreme reaction from her, sometimes even harshly grabbing Michael by the shoulders and shaking him. She felt terrible shame about her behavior, but in the heat of the moment had been unable to stop herself.

As the visit came to an end, I reflected back the story I had just heard of a stressful first few years with a challenging infant and of Angela's own emotional struggles. Now she and Michael were stuck in a pattern of daily head-to-head battles. I suggested that perhaps her guilt about her own behavior interfered with her ability to be present and enjoy her son. Angela nodded sadly.

When I saw Michael and his mother together the next week, Angela joyfully reported at the start of the visit that Michael had eaten an entire spaghetti dinner by himself. "I realized that he would eat when he's hungry!" I had not given any advice about what to do. By offering a safe space and an hour of nonjudgmental listening, I supported her efforts to listen to Michael. Relieved of those debilitating feelings of grief, guilt, and shame by sharing them with me, and identifying the source of her negative feelings, she found herself starting to enjoy time with him. Once he began to connect with her in more positive ways, he no longer needed to battle with her around eating. He reconnected with his own natural appetite.

Still the anxiety held a grip on Angela, who carried a brightly colored snack bag in to my office. "He didn't eat his lunch in school," she explained. But when she offered it to him, Michael, already involved in play, declined. I could see her body tense up, but she restrained herself for the whole visit. Then, as we were cleaning up, with only minutes left to the appointment, Michael said he wanted his snack, and more specifically, that he wanted to eat it now at the small table in my office. Angela looked questioningly at me. Although it might have meant the visit would run over by a few minutes, I nodded my consent. I felt that both mother and son wanted to share with me their pride in mastery of this important developmental step, also a first and meaningful step on a different path for their relationship.

When a recent study, widely publicized with such headlines as "Picky Eating in Children Linked to Anxiety, Depression and ADHD," showed an association between "selective eating" and what the authors termed "psychopathological symptoms," I saw another example of premature labeling of troubling behavior. Although picky eating can be a normal variation, as we see clearly in this story, and in many others throughout this book, restrictive eating patterns can be a communication of distress. Often eating behavior relates to both sensory sensitivities and issues in relationships. By exploring what the behavior means, we find the solution to the problem. If we simply name the behavior as a possible sign for a "disorder," we may miss that communication. Listening to both the child and the family offers an opportunity to set relationships on a healthy path. One might imagine that if Michael's issues had been addressed purely on a behavioral level, or labeled without listening to the story, Michael's relationship with food, and with his mother, might have become increasingly fraught.

Often a brief period of listening can create significant shifts in relationships. While I do not think every parent needs to see a specialist to raise a healthy child, I do think that every parent and child who is struggling needs to be heard. When both parent and child feel heard and recognized, there is profound joy in the reconnection that follows. For a young child whose brain is rapidly growing and changing, these changes can come quickly. For an older child, and when the suffering is deep, more time may be needed.

"Many of us have lost our capacity for listening and using loving speech in our families," writes Thich Nhat Hanh. "It may be no one is capable of listening to anyone else. So we feel very lonely even within our own families . . . listening like that is not to judge, to criticize, to condemn, or evaluate, but to listen with the single purpose of helping the other person suffer less."

Once parents have an opportunity to make sense of, or find meaning in, a child's behavior, what to do tends to follow naturally. The child's behavior is usually not a symptom of a disorder, but a form of communication. Understanding that communication reestablishes connection between parent and child.

A Call for Listening

My hope is that this book will support efforts, both by parents and professionals, to listen over time. Listening over time—weeks, months, years—offers the opportunity for children to grow into themselves.

The stories in this book come largely from my clinical experience. However, the importance of restoring the practice of listening goes well beyond issues related to therapy for children and families. Diagnostic labels and psychiatric drugs are symptoms of a cultural shift away from valuing human relationships. This has significance in realms of experience well beyond mental health care. Valuing space and time for listening has significance in families, schools, communities, and society as a whole. Abandoning listening has costs for all of us.

It is not simply a question of therapy vs. medication. It is about letting stories unfold. This is not a book against medication. Rather, it is meant to serve as a cautionary tale of what will happen if we neglect to listen to each other, and of the good that can come when we do protect the time and space for being present, for healing through relationships and human connection.

I will begin by showing the power of listening, and, in Chapter 2, the ways listening is being devalued. I will then show, in Chapter 3, how protecting space and time to listen to parents and children needs to begin in infancy, when the brain is most rapidly growing and changing. In early childhood, the brain makes as many as seven hundred connections per second. I will show how supporting new parents and babies will promote healthy development and resilience in the next generation. In Chapter 4 I will expand upon the notion that listening is a form of prevention. I will show how when we can listen early to children and parents, we can prevent progression to illness, and instead set development on a healthy path. In Chapter 5 I will show how valuing of the time itself, along with attention to the physical space, is essential to both prevention and effective healing. In Chapter 6 I will outline the factors, including influences of the health insurance and pharmaceutical industries, as well as pressures in the education system, that have let psychiatric diagnosis and medication replace listening. In Chapter 7 I will show how the social forces discouraging listening can be understood as a form of prejudice against children.

In the final section I will elaborate on different ways of listening that become open to us once we have protected the time and space. In Chapter 8 I will explore the importance of listening to the body. I will address the function of creativity in healing, both in terms of protecting space and time for a child's natural creativity to develop, as well as the creativity needed to help children whose behavior is off the beaten path. In Chapter 9 I'll elaborate on the way blocked mourning may underlie "behavior problems" in children. I will illustrate how healing occurs when parents have space and time to express and move through deep, often buried, feelings of grief. In conclusion, in Chapter 10 I'll show the dangers of certainty reflected in the ease with which diagnoses are made and medications are prescribed. I will contrast this with the value of tolerating uncertainty through the process of listening—of letting the story unfold from a position of wondering and not knowing.

Part One

An Endangered Art

One

On (Not) Giving Advice

D. W. Winnicott, pediatrician turned psychoanalyst, identified how parents (he refers to mothers because in the time he was writing, the mother was almost always the primary caregiver) naturally know what is right for their child. "No theory is acceptable that does not allow for the fact that mothers have always performed this essential function well enough." In an essay ironically titled "Advising Parents," he cautioned against the common practice of giving advice in the absence of the opportunity to hear the full story. Our "how-to" culture, with its abundance of "expert" advice, may itself be a barrier to listening, unintentionally undermining a parent's natural authority. Offering a prevailing contemporary perspective, a child psychiatrist at a major teaching hospital who was interviewing me for a radio show talked about the "parent training management" manual he had written. He argued that the parents "haven't been taught" and "don't know how to parent."

A preventive approach to children's mental health care recognizes the stresses on parents that may get in the way of their intuition. That stress takes many forms: the stress of a fussy baby; the everyday challenges of managing a family and work in today's fast-paced culture, often without the support of extended family; are frequent causes. Stress may come from more complex relational issues between parents, between siblings, between generations. It is not that they don't know how to parent, but that their natural abilities have been inhibited by stress, by negative models in the past, or both. Parents who say, "I don't want to raise Charlie the way I was raised" do not need "expert" advice. They need to develop confidence in their natural intuition. The goal is to support parents' efforts to find a way of raising their children that is in keeping with themselves, with each other, and with their child.

Like Winnicott, who said in his article, "I have no wish to carry this attitude to absurd lengths," I do recognize that guidance from a person more experienced and knowledgeable may at times be very useful for parents. In many cultures, grandmothers fill this role. In American culture, many mothers do not choose this route. Journalist Jennifer Senior describes how, in researching her book *All Joy and No Fun: The Paradox of Modern Parenthood,* when she asked parents where they went for advice, no parents named their own mothers. There may be a range of explanations for this phenomenon, but when these relationships are fraught, or when grandmothers are far away or no longer living, this source of guidance may not even be available. One colleague, a preschool teacher and gymnastics coach, suggested the word "coach." She explained how a coach supports an athlete in being the best he can be given his unique set of traits, without dictating a set formula for success. The trouble comes from advising, coaching, and guiding in the absence of space and time for hearing the full story.

Parents in my office often sound like they are riding on a see-saw, moving from the worry "It's my fault" to the fear "There is something wrong with him." Well-intentioned reassurance can have the opposite effect when parents quickly move to "Then there must be something wrong with *me*." Feelings of guilt alternate with fear, even panic. They worry that the struggles the family is experiencing are somehow a reflection of them as "bad" parents.

I have found that Winnicott's the concept of the "good-enough mother" helps support parents as they make efforts to set relationships on a different path. This "good-enough" parent is present, but not perfect. In fact, it is the very imperfections in parents that promote healthy development. They offer the growing child the experience of surviving disruptions, paving the way for managing life's inevitable disappointments. Winnicott writes:

> The good-enough "mother" (not necessarily the infant's own mother) is one who makes active adaptation to the infant's needs, an active adaptation that gradually lessens according to the infant's growing ability to . . . tolerate the results of frustration . . . *If all goes well* the infant can actually come to gain from the experience of frustration.

A hefty dose of guilt, and with that a tendency to feel blamed, naturally comes with the role of parent. A label for the child may ease that guilt. But when parents resist diagnostic labels, they may be described as being in denial. This negative language sets up relationships of antagonism. Framed in a more positive, empowering light, a feeling of guilt may translate to a sense of responsibility. "I'm guilty" can also mean "I'm responsible." Being listened to without judgment moves parents from helplessness to responsible action.

I have treated hundreds of families for whom this kind of listening has led to significant shifts in development and to new levels of connection and communication. However, sometimes after setting out on this path to discover meaning, a family will not return.

While in each individual case I may not know the reason, there are some recurring themes. It may be that if the disruptions have occurred over many years, the concept of the "good-enough mother" is not sufficient to neutralize the guilt. Often social pressures, from family, friends, teachers, and others, to diagnose a disorder overwhelm parents and so do not allow for this patient exploration. Sometimes years later I learn that that the parents have divorced. A "problem" child may have been hiding a troubled marriage. I may have, in the face of parents who wish to know what to do, given advice before I understood the full story. Or we may have been too quick to explore deeply painful, long-buried issues.

Listening for the True Self

> The story of a human being does not start at five years or two, or at six months, but starts at birth—and before birth if you like; and each baby is from the start a person, and needs to be known by someone. No one can know a baby as well as the baby's own mother can.
>
> —D. W. Winnicott

When parents worry whether there is "something wrong with my child," I try to reframe the question, drawing on another central concept of Winnicott's, the "true self." When the "good-enough mother" recognizes her child's experience and helps him make sense of it, his true self begins to emerge. Stress, fear, guilt, and issues from other relationships may get in the way of that recognition, of understanding his behavior in the context of his unique strengths and vulnerabilities.

Instead of joining the parents in looking for "what's wrong," I suggest to them that we take some time to think about why the child might be behaving as he does, why his behavior might make sense from his perspective. I have found that with this opportunity to be heard, and in turn to listen to what their child is communicating, most parents prefer not to have their child labeled with a disorder.

A big roadblock, however, is set up by our health-care and education systems. These may push parents in the direction of labeling by requiring a diagnosis to obtain services. There is often a frenzied need to give a name to a problem so as to feel that something is being done. In all of the stories I tell in this book, treatment is definitely needed. It is important not to fall in to the trap of thinking that if a child does not have a disorder, families don't need help. The "disease" vs. "normal" split is inaccurate and potentially harmful. In my practice I get around this problem by diagnosing almost everyone with the nonspecific "adjustment reaction." I then bill for the number of minutes spent in counseling that in reality is mostly listening. One reader commented on my blog, "I hope that by giving them time and space to listen this doesn't mean a delay in treatment." We have lost sight of the fact that, especially for a developing child and his family, listening can be the treatment.

In his wise book *Far from the Tree*, Andrew Solomon explores the process of acceptance for families who have children with a wide range of differences. He speaks to the need to strive toward strength and healing by constructing meaning. Unfortunately, both our health-care and education systems force parents and professionals in the opposite direction by requiring that something be "wrong" with a child for us to be able to pay attention.

The story of Mary and Liam offers an example of offering space and time to support a mother's efforts to recognize her child's experience and reach what Winnicott would call his true self. Mary was convinced that her three-month-old son, Liam, was autistic.

She felt she couldn't connect with him. Her third child, he was remarkably different from his older brothers, now three and six years old. They had both been colicky in the early months, but had grown into active boys with a lot to say. Liam, in contrast, was quiet from the moment he was born. He hardly even cried in the delivery room. Despite the doctor's reassurances, Mary wondered from those first moments if there was something "wrong with him." As the weeks went on, not only was he quiet, but he also seemed to her not to be connected. She would put her face up close to his and try to engage him to look at her face and follow. But she was rarely successful. As the weeks went on, her efforts intensified while her anxiety escalated.

With a full hour together, we sat on the floor and observed Liam together. I noticed right away that my attempts to engage him by talking to him and looking in to his face were met by a rather remote expression. He appeared to be looking past me, perhaps at the lights on the ceiling, but it wasn't clear. I saw Mary's rising alarm. Resisting a similar reaction in myself, I said, "Let's give it time."

Liam lay on a blanket on the floor, at first continuing his seemingly random scanning of the room. I spoke quietly to him, noticing how he was sticking out his tongue. I imitated his movements and gradually he began to engage. Mary noticed that he seemed to be responding to my mirroring of his expression. We observed a gradual yet remarkable transformation. In the quiet calm of this space, so dramatically different from the normal chaos of his everyday life, he seemed to come out of his shell. It started with a smile, at first seemingly random, but then clearly in response to my smile. Mary continued to speak with him in a soft voice but, following my example, rather than putting her face up close to him, she spoke in a more natural way as part of our conversation. Liam became increasingly animated. Mary and I noticed, with rising joy and relief, that not only was he fixing on and following his mother's face, but he was cooing in a responsive conversation with her. He kicked his legs and moved his arms in an expression of increasing delight.

Marveling at this little baby's extraordinary capacity for communication, we wondered whether his quiet nature was part of an extreme sensitivity to the relentless sensory input from a busy household with two older brothers. Perhaps he was adapting by tuning out. He was in fact very engaged, but he preferred a quiet voice that was not "in his face." He was finding his own way in the world.

What had happened between Mary and Liam was a kind of miscommunication, a dance of stepped-on toes. The less he connected, the more her attempts to engage him intensified. An illness model that places a problem squarely in the child leads us to miss opportunities for growth and healing. The "problem" was neither in Mary nor in Liam. They just needed to learn a new dance. With the help of a quiet space and time to listen, Mary could recognize that her well-meaning efforts might have been experienced as intrusive, given Liam's sensitivity. As her anxiety grew and her efforts to engage Liam intensified, he withdrew further.

Relief flooded Mary, but her anxiety did not let go. Had she caused him harm by missing his cues? I pointed out how easy it had been for us to engage Liam. He was ready to communicate. Clearly, Mary had been doing something right. Research supporting Winnicott's concept of the "good-enough mother" has shown that even when parents miss an infant's cues in 70 percent of interactions, as long as these misses are recognized and repaired, development moves forward in a healthy way.

When I saw them together a month later, she spoke joyfully of the fun the family was having with Liam, who had developed into an engaged and happy baby. Now, taking a few minutes every day to have some quiet time with him, she fell deeper and deeper in love. She marveled at his individuality even at the tender age of four months. This "disruption" led to new levels of intimacy between Mary and her son.

Stories: A Path to the True Self

When I was a medical student, I had the privilege of sitting in on a child development class taught to child psychiatry fellows at Cornell Medical Center by the late Paulina Kernberg, a gifted child psychiatrist and analyst. One of the fellows brought his nine-month-old son as a subject. I vividly recall witnessing the joy of his accomplishments. I saw child development as a wonder of nature that unfolds with purpose and clarity.

When a child struggles without progress, whether in infancy, adolescence, or somewhere in between, that developmental path has somehow become derailed. Continuing the metaphor, to get a train back on track requires going back to the beginning. It requires telling the story from the start, to make sense of where and how it got derailed. Only then can development begin to go forward in a healthy direction. Listening offers the opportunity to tell the story, and to have the story heard, from the beginning.

Development is the child's story. Storytelling is equally important for parents. A person might have a narrative of his life that makes sense to him, only to have it completely upended when a child comes in to the world. A different narrative is formed that includes a new individual with unique qualities and needs. Relationships both between parents as well as with each individual parent's past may be significantly altered in this developmental stage of parenthood.

The frenzy of activity that parenthood entails often leaves little time for reflection. By the time there is a "behavior problem," be it colic, sleep problems, separation anxiety, explosive behavior, or any number of issues that young families contend with, parents may be so focused on just getting through the day that there is no time to make sense of what is happening. The stage is set for the appealing array of advice about what to do that our culture offers to parents. Yet taking time to tell that story may in fact be the solution to the problem.

Supporting a child's healthy development calls for an ability to remain calm; to respond to what is happening in real time, without letting your own history interfere. When the way a child's behavior echoes past experiences is out of your awareness, this kind of response may not be possible. Knowing your own story can make it possible for you to be present with your child in a way that allows his or her true self to emerge.

How Listening Promotes Knowledge

Listening has evolutionary significance. Knowledge about what is needed for survival is transmitted from one generation to the next. The ability to understand one's own and others' behavior as a reflection of underlying feelings is a uniquely human quality that allows for this transmission of knowledge. When children feel heard and understood, they develop what psychoanalyst Peter Fonagy has termed "epistemic trust." *Epistemic* means "of or relating to knowledge." He defines the concept as "an individual's willingness to consider new knowledge from another person as trustworthy, generalizable, and relevant." In other words, the way we acquire new knowledge about ourselves, others, and the world around us is intimately intertwined with how we are listened to as a developing child. Children learn, from the cues a trusted caregiver offers, to whom they should listen and what is important for them to learn. They develop the ability to think not only about their own feelings and behavior, but also to understand the motivations and intentions of others.

Being listened to, or held in mind, is thus of central importance if children are to manage in increasingly complex social environments. Flexibility in thinking, and with that openness to new ideas, goes hand in hand with the early experience of being heard. In contrast, when children grow up without this openness and trust, they may be closed off to new information. A lack of knowledge and skills may be perpetuated from one generation to the next.

Decades before Fonagy, John Bowlby was among the first to identify the evolutionary significance of our earliest relationships, as he describes in his book *A Secure Base*. Capturing the essence of what many would agree we want for our own children and for the next generation, he writes that a child who is held and heard in this way is likely to "become increasingly self-reliant and bold in his exploration of the world, co-operative with others, and also—a very important point—sympathetic and helpful to others in distress."

Two

Listening Devalued

In the context of rising reports of depression and suicide in college, one student described a school administrator's coming to visit her in the hospital following a second suicide attempt. He asked, "Are we going to make this a pattern?" and then handed her his business card.

In another example from my practice, a parent described calling the emergency student support services when she was worried about her son Evan's emotional state during his first semester at college. After a five-minute conversation, she was told by the person who responded to her call, "We can make an appointment with the psychiatrist to see if he needs medication."

Significant forces in our society work against listening. These forces come into play when a parent, whose child may be struggling with a range of issues, comes in contact with a system of care that offers only behavior management, parent training, and increasingly diagnostic labels and medication. These forms of treatment may crowd out space and time for listening.

Psychiatric medication may be useful and necessary when a person is unable to function without it. In cases of severely out-of-control behaviors and emotions, medication can offer symp-tomatic relief. In certain circumstances, it may even be lifesaving. It may make other forms of therapy possible, including relationship-based therapies and self-regulating activities, such as yoga, music, or meditation. But that is not the way these medications are being used. Because they can be so effective at eliminating distress in the short term, they are very appealing, almost irresistible, as a single solution in our fast-paced, quick-fix culture.

A 2013 CDC (Centers for Disease Control and Prevention) survey reported that close to 50 percent of adolescents who have taken psychiatric medication in the past month have not seen a mental health professional in the past year. It suggests that we are becoming comfortable with medicating away feelings, without op-portunity to gain the insight and understanding that are central to true healing and continued growth.

Controversy swirls around the subject of psychiatric medica-tion, in both adults and children, not only of antidepressants, but also stimulants and increasingly antipsychotics. "Are the medica-tions useful?" "What is the role of the placebo effect?" "What are the long-term side effects?" "Should we blame the drug compa-nies?" Marcia Angell, former editor of the *New England Journal of Medicine*, grappled with these issues in a series of articles in the *New York Review of Books*, concluding:

> Our reliance on psychoactive drugs, seemingly for all of life's discontents, *tends to close off other options* (italics mine.) In view of the risks and questionable long-term effectiveness of drugs, we need to do better.

Angell calls on us to "rethink the care of troubled children." The question of using psychoactive drugs in children is fundamentally different and on a greater order of magnitude than with adults. It goes beyond the relative merits of psychotherapy or medication, or even of the potentially serious side effects. As Angell says, the problem lies in what is *not* done when psychiatric medication is used to treat children.

Blocking the Path to Resilience

In my first book, *Keeping Your Child in Mind*, I describe the extensive research showing how children become capable of emotional regulation and overall mental health when those who care for them respond to the meaning of their behavior, rather than the behavior itself. Children develop resilience when their struggles are acknowledged—but not erased—through the inevitable stresses of life. When, however, starting at a young age, rather than learning to handle stress in the context of supportive relationships, a child's "symptoms" are "managed" or increasingly medicated away, the areas of the brain responsible for emotional regulation may not develop properly. The brain is actually wired through relationships. The areas of the brain responsible for emotional regulation develop when children's immature abilities are regulated together with a trusted caregiver who understands what they are feeling.

If, as the challenges of life increase, dosages are simply increased in strength and complexity, often with added diagnoses, children may learn to be defined by their disorder and by their medication. It is not uncommon for children in preadolescence and even younger to be diagnosed and started on medication that is then continued despite ongoing massive developmental changes. The control of behavior with medication may then continue to interfere with these children's emerging sense of self.

In a course she teaches entitled "Keeping the Brain in Mind," Francine Lapides referred to psychotherapists as "neuroarchitects." In a relationship with a therapist who is carefully listening, fully attuned to the patient's feelings, the patient's brain may actually change, in turn changing the way that person responds to stress. The changed biochemistry of the brain may actually help a person learn to think about feelings and manage difficult experiences.

Parents are the original neuroarchitects. When a child is struggling, whether with sadness, anxiety, or explosive behavior, a parent's "presence of mind" helps that child to make sense of and manage his own strong emotions. Parents themselves need to feel supported so as to recognize what their child is experiencing, and be with their child in a way that promotes healthy emotional development.

The Rising Use of Psychiatric Medication

The widespread use of medication has fundamentally changed the landscape of mental health care. We condone their use alone, without concurrent relationship-based treatments. A recent study documented that pediatricians, who diagnose and treat the majority of cases of ADHD, use medication without any psychosocial support in close to 90 percent of patients.

When medications can be used this way, in the absence of time for relationship-based treatment, the professionals who offer opportunity for listening and human connection are devalued, both culturally and monetarily. Such attitudes and financial disincentives decrease the availability of qualified professionals.

Pediatricians, whose long-standing relationships with children and families makes them ideally suited for preventive interventions, are discouraged from using their time to listen. In our current reimbursement system, a practice will better survive financially when primary care clinicians see four to six children in an hour, rather than spend one hour listening to one family, even though, as we will see throughout this book, an hour of listening can have great preventive value.

Social workers, psychologists, and others who offer relationship-based treatment in which feelings can be recognized and understood are reimbursed less and less by insurance companies. At the same time, they are required by the health insurance industry to exert increasing effort, jumping through an increasing number of hoops, leading many not to participate in insurance plans. Families struggle to find a qualified clinician who accepts their insurance. Thus the drugs themselves, because they can replace people, become inextricably linked with the shortage of quality mental health care. With fewer qualified professionals to do the work of listening, those who remain are overwhelmed. Finding help from people with time and space to be present in a way that promotes healing grows harder and harder.

Evan had been a patient in my practice for many years when I received that call from his mother about her conversation with the college emergency support services. He had always had a tendency to be anxious, but it was not a significant problem for him until he applied to college. He was struggling with this developmental step. But rather than prescribe medication, I referred him to a therapist. I was fortunate to have an excellent colleague who had time and took his insurance. She helped him make sense of his fears.

During a rough patch in the winter of that first year away, following that disturbing call, his mother filled me in. Knowing that confidentiality prevented me from talking about my relationship with Evan, his parents simply wanted to talk about their experience. They told me they had discovered that in his moments of distress when they simply stayed on the phone, containing their own worries and need to "fix" the problem, being present with him, rather than jumping in to offer advice, they would observe a significant transformation. Their son's breathing would gradually slow, he would become calm, and he would again be able to think clearly.

I spoke with Evan following that first year away at college. He came home for the summer feeling positively triumphant. He had done well academically. But most important, he had struggled through a difficult time and come through to the other side. He was positively joyful with this newfound strength. The listening of his therapist, his parents, and myself, both to Evan and to his parents, offered Evan the opportunity to heal and to grow.

As parents, it's easy for us to panic when our child struggles. The wish to "do something before it's too late" comes from a place of deep love and identification. However, if we can pause and slow down, through careful listening we can set the child on a healthy path. For Evan's parents during some of the worst late-night phone calls, it was difficult not to panic, to fear that there was "something wrong with him." That voice of the emergency worker suggesting they send him to a psychiatrist for medication evaluation echoed in their mind. But they sought help from friends, family, and from each other. They created what Winnicott termed a "holding environment" for themselves, in which their own feelings could be recognized and contained. In turn they could offer a space for Evan to struggle and eventually connect with his own strengths.

While Lapides correctly points out that listening can change the brain in long-term psychotherapy with adults, these kinds of changes are far easier to make in a child, when the brain is rapidly growing and changing. But when symptoms are treated with medication alone, the opportunity to change a child's brain by supporting relationships may be lost. The problem is less one of overmedication than of underlistening.

Evan's story reflects the essence of resilience. There were times, especially very late at night, when Evan's parents would lose their cool. When they had gotten some sleep and had a chance to re-group, they would be open with Evan about how they had felt, sharing with him that they had not been at their best, while setting limits on late-night phone calls and protecting time to talk when they could all think more clearly. Evan had safe, secure relation-ships with people who didn't try to fix everything but stayed with him as he worked through his fears. He came not only to name his feelings but also to connect with a new sense of himself.

With pills so easily available without opportunity for insight or understanding, Evan might have taken a different path. In the short term, it might have been easier than struggling with the pain of separation. He might have done equally well academically, but his success would be tied intimately with a pill, without a space for discovering meaning. It was the struggle itself that led to new strength and growth.

How Labels Preclude Listening

A number of years ago I went to a talk given by a local "ADHD expert" to a group of pediatricians. The aim of the talk was to guide us in doing ADHD evaluations, given the time constraints of pri-mary care practice. "It's all about the rating scales," he said. "You need to train your staff to give out the right scales. The key to working kids up is getting the scales done ahead of time. Nothing happens in the office." This doctor proudly displayed his version of the main rating scale, the Vanderbilt, which he had divided into two time slots, because "kids have different symptoms at

different times of day." Evaluation and treatment of ADHD in pediatric practices, where the majority of these diagnoses are made,
consists primarily of scoring rating scales, making a decision to use
medication, and once the decision is made, having follow-up visits
every three months to adjust medication dose according to symptoms and side effects.

I began to develop my views on this subject of diagnostic labeling and psychiatric medication when, after practicing general pediatrics for close to twenty years, I inherited an "ADHD practice"
from a wonderful man, a larger-than-life, toss-babies-in-the-air
pediatrician with a hearty laugh. He never had an unkind word to
say about anyone. He had retired from general pediatrics and was
only seeing "ADHD patients," when he died suddenly in a tragic
accident. His patients were devastated. My colleagues asked if I
would take over his practice. Out of loyalty to him, I agreed.

I learned that he was seeing his 170 or so patients once every
three to six months for a thirty-minute visit. This was pretty much
the standard of care in pediatrics. But I felt that if I were going
to prescribe psychiatric medication to these children, I wanted to
learn what was going on in their lives. I had the good fortune to be
simultaneously studying psychoanalysis and contemporary developmental science at the Berkshire Psychoanalytic Institute. This
experience was opening my mind to the value of time and space
for listening.

I particularly tried to open things up when kids were doing
poorly. For example, I didn't just focus on adjusting the dose of
medication when they were failing in school, but explored other
possible reasons for their academic struggles. This meant uncover-
ing some pretty difficult problems, including complex family conflict. Some families got angry and left. "We thought you just weighed
and measured Johnny and then refilled the prescription."

However, it was not uncommon for a parent, given that space and time, to reveal a critical and unexpected piece of information, often toward the very end of the visit. A kindergarten teacher referred five-year-old Max to me, suggesting to his parents that he might need medication. His behavior had been disruptive since preschool, but was now affecting his ability to learn. There was concern that he might not be able to move on to first grade. With standardized forms already filled out by his parents and his teacher in anticipation of an ADHD evaluation, the question being asked of me was: would he meet diagnostic criteria, and if so, would medication be indicated?

I met with Max's parents, Cynthia and Rob, who described classic symptoms of ADHD, including prolonged battles at home around such simple tasks as getting dressed for school. About halfway through the visit, I began to ask about past history. "How was your pregnancy with him?" There was a pause, during which the parents exchanged looks. "Actually, I'm not his biological mother," said Cynthia.

Now it was my turn to pause. I was shocked to receive this important piece of information so late in the evaluation process. With some reluctance, Cynthia and Rob went on to tell me that Max's birth mother, Rob's ex-wife, was seriously mentally ill, had been only intermittently involved in his life, and had disappeared completely two years earlier. But, they assured me, Max never talked about his mother and it wasn't an important issue.

"If you ask questions you get answers—and hardly anything else." This well-known aphorism in medicine comes from a book, *The Doctor, His Patient and the Illness* by Hungarian psychiatrist Michael Balint. In his work with groups of primary care doctors in post–World War II London, where many patients had symptoms related to complex psychological trauma, Balint supported their efforts to use themselves as the treatment. He writes, "The discussion quickly revealed . . . that by far the most frequently used drug in general practice was the doctor himself." Balint encouraged these physicians to be fully present to listen to their patients, rather than asking questions guided only by a need to make a diagnosis.

I agreed that medication might be helpful for Max. Whatever the cause of the behavior, stimulant medication can, in the short term, be very effective at decreasing symptoms of inattentiveness and hyperactivity. However, building on the trust his parents had developed with me as their pediatrician, I suggested that the loss of his mother was a very important issue that needed to be addressed. They accepted my referral to a therapist. I was fortunate to have an excellent colleague who accepted their insurance. He wisely explained to them that children do grieve, and engaged the whole family in working with him around this painful but important task.

The very structure of the DSM (*Diagnostic and Statistical Manual of Mental Disorders*), the "bible of psychiatry" and primary tool currently used for making psychiatric diagnoses, can preclude listening. It creates a kind of circular reasoning by defining disorders by symptoms and then in indicating that if a patient has this set of symptoms, she has that disorder. Our current system of mental health care, by emphasizing the "what" rather than "why," captures only the behavior, but not what the behavior is communicating.

A recent publication by the American Psychiatric Association that assesses clinicians' knowledge about the new *DSM 5* (the latest version of this "bible") exemplifies this problem. Using two vignettes, one of a sixty-five-year-old woman with increasing fears of leaving the house, and the other a thirty-five-year-old man who has developed a fear of flying, the book introduces current categories for diagnosing anxiety. Listing these, including the newest "social anxiety disorder," the book asks readers to choose the "cause" of these individuals' anxiety. In another example of circular reasoning, the symptom defines the label and the label is then taken as the cause.

This whole approach is driving mental health professionals away from listening. Psychologist Jonathan Shedler describes asking a fourth-year psychiatry resident, after she has presented a case, what they are treating the patient for. The resident answers, "Generalized anxiety disorder." But when Shedler asks the doctor in training what her patient is anxious about, he gets a blank look. To his question of how she understands her patient's anxiety psychologically, he gets this response: "I don't think it's psychological, I think it's biological." This way of thinking leaves no room for hearing the patient's story, for finding meaning in her behavior.

Symptom management and the prescribing of psychiatric medication without opportunity to discover the cause of a child's anxiety can be a direct obstacle to unfolding that child's sense of self. Yet when this approach, in children as young as four, is condoned and increasingly common, and powerful medications, at least in the short term, have eliminated the "symptom," supporting parents' efforts to explore the meaning of their child's anxiety is very difficult.

While studying for my recertification exam as required by the American Board of Pediatrics, using the review course offered by the American Academy of Pediatrics (AAP), I came across a question asking about treatment for a seven-year-old girl with separation anxiety. The case described problems since preschool, bedtime resistance, and frequent tantrums. Her parents were divorced and she was an only child. At her father's house she expressed fear that something would happen to her mother.

The "correct" answer was cognitive behavioral therapy (CBT) to "work on skills for managing her distress." Prescribing an SSRI

(selective serotonin reuptake inhibitor), such as Prozac, was recommended as a second line of treatment. Play therapy in which
a therapist would "assist the child in recognizing the cause" was
incorrect.

When I wrote about this experience in a blog post, many readers came to the defense of "evidence-based" CBT (cognitive behavioral therapy). One wrote in a comment that the assessment
portion of the treatment would offer the opportunity to learn the
story. But, I replied, that is an example of putting the cart before
the horse. CBT or even medication might have a role to play, but
how do we know if we do not first take time to hear the full story?

What might be some possible causes of her anxiety? Is her
mother depressed? Her father? Is there substance abuse in either
parent? Did she observe conflict, perhaps even violence, between
her parents in the years preceding their divorce? Is there a family history of anxiety, suggesting a genetic vulnerability? Does
she have sensory processing challenges that cause her to be overwhelmed in the stimulating classroom? Some combination of all of
these factors might exist.

Perhaps the mother of the child in the vignette had similar
struggles with anxiety as a child. But rather than being met with
understanding, she received a slap across the face. She may be terrified that her daughter will suffer as she did. If she is flooded with
stress due to her daughter's behavior, she might, without thinking,
lash out. Or more likely, as her maternal instinct to protect her
child overrides a rage response, she might shut down emotionally.
Either way, her child will be alone with these difficult feelings.
When we teach children "skills" to "manage" feelings and behavior, without first listening for the meaning, the story may be buried. It may emerge years later, sometimes in the form of serious
mental illness.

One eight-year-old girl who had been diagnosed with anxiety disorder by her previous pediatrician was brought to me to get her prescription refilled. After several hour-long appointments, some with her alone and some with her mother, I learned that, like the child in the vignette, she had divorced parents. During her every-other weekend visits with her father, he drank heavily, leaving her to care for her two younger brothers. The primary problem needing treatment was his alcoholism. My patient's behavior represented an adaptive response to a frightening situation.

Where in the treatment plan recommended by the AAP is there opportunity to uncover such a story? Parents may experience terrible shame about their own behavior. Parents share this kind of information only when they feel safe. Safety comes when there is time and space for nonjudgmental listening. When parents can make sense of their child's behavior, they are in an ideal position to support that child in managing her unique vulnerabilities. When they themselves feel strong and supported, parents are best suited to provide a kind of cognitive behavioral therapy. This requires bringing into awareness the way their child's behavior may provoke their own difficult feelings, and in a sense moving these feelings out of the way. They can help their child to name feelings, identify provocative situations, and develop strategies to manage these experiences. It is the responsibility of the parent, not the child, to make sense of and find meaning in the behavior. The experience of anxiety is then incorporated into that child's emerging sense of self in a healthy way.

Thinking of Evan, his anxiety was a normal reaction to the task of separation, magnified by his natural tendency to be anxious. It would become a disorder only if he could not manage, or regulate, his anxiety. When he could calm down in the quiet presence of his parents on the other end of the phone, the thinking parts of his brain would come back on line. Rather than being overwhelmed, he could name the feeling and move through and then past it.

Silencing Communication

Perhaps the most serious effect of labels and medication is the silencing of a generation of children. When I took over my colleague's "ADHD practice," I saw many children who had been diagnosed with ADHD and treated for many years without any significant exploration of their family situation. One mother told me about her own struggles with untreated depression. Another spoke of her recent recovery from drug addiction and the child's father's recent deployment to Iraq. A third child quietly told his mother he was frightened when she pulled his hair and hit him. The effects of these experiences on the child were unrecognized and unaddressed. Without offering time for listening, we do not hear these stories.

I thought about this devaluing of listening when I reviewed my son's high school essay on *To Kill a Mockingbird*. I was surprised and pleased to rediscover, or perhaps discover for the first time now that I was viewing it from the perspective of over fifty years of life experience, the profound wisdom of the book.

In one of the novel's most famous quotes, Atticus tells his daughter, Scout, "You never really understand a person until you consider things from his point of view, until you climb in his skin and walk around in it." I now understand this as a description of an essential human characteristic, namely the ability to reflect on the meaning of another person's behavior. Psychoanalyst Peter Fonagy argues, in a way similar to John Bowlby's representation of attachment behavior, that this ability to find meaning has evolutionary significance and is important for survival.

I wonder whether we are losing this essential human capacity. We no longer value taking the time and space to think about the meaning of behavior. We aim simply to name it and, if it is causing disruption, eliminate it. The most common phrases I hear from parents who come to my office with concerns of behavior problems are "she never listens," followed by "tell me what to do to make her listen." The problem may indeed be not listening, but it is the adults who are not listening to the children or to each other. In our fast-paced, technology-driven age, we rarely take the time to put ourselves in another person's skin.

When Scout comes home from her first day of school, upset with her teacher, her father tells her that she's new, too. When he does, he helps Scout to understand her teacher's perhaps impatient behavior from a different point of view, to appreciate that the teacher herself may have been stressed and overwhelmed.

Time in the clinician's office is measured in minutes. But development is measured in years. We will never go back to the slow pace depicted in the 1960 novel, with its large expanses of time to listen. But we need to be very careful not to give it up completely. For if putting oneself in another person's skin is an essential part of our humanity, we need to be careful to protect the needed space and time.

Part Two

Listening in Practice

Three

Listening to Babies

Three-month-old Haley changed my life. Crying almost non-stop, she had been treated unsuccessfully for colic by multiple doctors, with formula changes and medication trials. Her mother, Nicole, had been diagnosed with postpartum depression and was being treated by her primary care physician, who, in the face of her steady decline, had offered to increase her dose of antidepressant medication. A colleague referred the family to me.

We had a full hour and a spacious office. Haley announced herself with the relentless insistent screaming that only young infants can do. Her exhausted father, Dan, feeling helpless in the face of his wife's despair, held the baby while pacing the floor.

Nicole collapsed on the couch, her body shaking with sobs of defeat. Through her tears she told me her story. I remember one striking detail all these years later. The day before she had been carrying groceries and an apple fell out of the bag. Nicole had folded to the ground weeping. But through the blur of sleep deprivation, Nicole realized that she did not want to miss out on this time in her daughter's life in a drugged haze. She longed to find a way to connect.

Gradually as she spoke, her sobs slowed down. In parallel, Haley's relentless crying began to decrease in intensity. Nicole told me a bit about herself, her family, her pregnancy, and Haley's first three months. When she was eleven years old she had been placed on Prozac for anxiety. Many years and medication changes later, she found herself unable to get off an SSRI when she wanted to get pregnant. She tried again after she conceived, but the symptoms of anxiety returned in greater intensity, so she resigned herself to staying on the medication. Nicole described her pregnancy as stressful. Haley had been "like this" from the moment she was born. The nurses brought her back within minutes of taking her to the nursery—unable to console her. She was quiet only in her mother's arms. In the weeks since they had gotten home, things had only become worse.

Toward the end of our visit a quiet calm descended. We were able to sit on the floor and observe Haley, who was awake and alert. She cooed at her mother, whose relief and joy were palpable. But when Dan sneezed, Haley was startled. Her arms flew over her head in a primitive "moro" reflex, and her screaming resumed. Nicole swaddled her and walked around, explaining how these kinds of disruptions were making sleep impossible. But now we could clearly see that this sensitivity to sounds and rapid descent into screaming resided in Haley. Fortified by the nurses' observations, and for the first time taking in the fact that the crying was not her "fault," Nicole relaxed. She felt a calm come over her as some of the debilitating feelings of guilt and inadequacy began to subside. I gave no advice about what to do. Recognizing her vulnerable emotional state, I did give her the names of some psychotherapists, and we scheduled an appointment for the following week.

When she and Haley arrived at the door to my office for that appointment, I observed a remarkable transformation. I was struck by being in the presence of two people in love. Haley cooed and joyfully kicked her legs as Nicole smiled with delight, cooing in response. When Nicole was finally able to shift her attention to say hello to me, she told me, "I feel like Haley's just been born." I asked her how she made sense of the change. "I felt you heard me," she said. "And Dan did, too. For the first time he really understood what I was feeling."

She had made an appointment with the psychotherapist but hadn't yet been. She decided not to increase her dose of medication. She had, however, let Dan watch Haley while she went to a yoga class. She could make sense of Haley's behavior in light of her sensitivity to sounds and the chaotic reaction brought on by her startle reflex. Rather than falling apart along with Haley, at these moments she would make use of her yoga skills to breathe through them and stay calm. The effort required in helping Haley settle seemed to lessen.

That first hour, when Dan listened to Nicole, Nicole and Dan listened to Haley, and I listened to all three, had offered an opportunity for profound connection, setting the whole family in a new direction.

Over the coming months, I saw them intermittently, as they had had a rough start and some extra time was useful. But then they continued seeing their general pediatrician. By the time Haley was a year old, Nicole felt strong and confident. Soon she was pregnant with her second child.

A Missed Opportunity

The dramatic contrast between this hopeful encounter, that seemed to alter this young family's life path, and the rest of the appointments in my practice that, in keeping with the standard of care in pediatrics, consisted primarily of writing refills for medications, led me to conclude that this practice was not right. The experience provided the motivation for me to want to do things differently.

As the behavioral pediatrics specialist in a general pediatrics practice, most of my visits were for ADHD evaluation. As I have described, the expectation was that, based on a standardized checklist and history of symptoms, I would determine whether a child had the diagnosis, and if so, decide whether or not to prescribe medication.

When a number of years earlier I shifted within the same setting from general pediatrics to practice behavioral pediatrics exclusively, the most significant change was the length of the visits—from fifteen to thirty minutes to a full hour. Rather than rely primarily on a symptom checklist, I had time to listen to the story. In almost every case, most of which were scheduled as an "ADHD evaluation," whether the child was 3, 7, 11, or even 17, parents would offer variations of the statement "He's been like this since birth." Recent longitudinal research has indeed identified a close link between behavioral dysregulation in infancy—defined as excessive crying, feeding, and sleep difficulties—and behavioral problems in childhood and adolescence.

I began to notice that I was hearing Haley's story, only years later, with a legion of missed opportunities in between. Problems went unrecognized and unaddressed. Many of these parents had struggled terribly for a long time. Often it started with depression and/ or anxiety in pregnancy or in the postpartum period. With severe sleep deprivation, marital stress, and other factors contributing to problems of emotional regulation, fussy babies had developed into difficult toddlers. Transitions to preschool were fraught. Pediatricians, under the time constraint of the fifteen- to thirty-minute visit, could not hear about such things as marital conflict, parental mental illness, or substance abuse, much less take the time needed to make an appropriate referral. They could only offer brief advice, generic parent guidance, and other forms of instruction in what to do.

Often years of behavior management had failed and now these children, entering the structured school system, were "disruptive," "impulsive," "distracted." They fell into categories matching *DSM* criteria for ADHD. Teachers recommended ADHD evaluations. With no opportunity to explore the developmental underpinnings of these issues, children were diagnosed and medicated. A pill, effective in the short term, transformed these "difficult" children into compliant students who could now "sit still and learn." But these improvements were often short lived, and years of medication adjustments followed. Other unintended consequences followed as well. At the time I saw Haley and Nicole, we were beginning to see an explosion in the number of high school students abusing these very stimulants that we were prescribing in huge quantities.

I found myself longing to see more infant-mother pairs like Haley and Nicole—to be able to help set things right from the beginning. When I took the time to get a detailed family and developmental history for children being evaluated for ADHD, in almost every case we could trace the roots of these problems back to early childhood. When we could make sense of the meaning of the behavior in a developmental context, we could begin, as I will discuss in more detail in the next chapter and Part 4, to think creatively about solutions. But once a child was in school, forces leading to diagnosis and medication were great, and resources and time for careful listening sorely lacking.

Opportunities to prevent these problems lay in listening to the very earliest relationships. I was fortunate to be able to pursue these opportunities through the University of Massachusetts Boston Infant-Parent Mental Health program created by developmental psychologist Ed Tronick. There I was exposed to leading research in this new and growing discipline. For intensive monthly three-day weekends, we learned directly from the researchers themselves. Equally important, I was able to learn side by side with colleagues from a wide range of disciplines who recognized and understood the value of working with infants and parents to prevent later problems. We shared a passion for protecting and nurturing these earliest relationships. While many pediatricians and psychiatrists coming out of medical schools are trained to identify and treat illness and disease, these colleagues offered a new perspective, with a focus on identifying strength and resilience.

The work of British researchers Lynne Murray and Peter Cooper introduced me to a wealth of evidence supporting my clinical observation of the association between postpartum depression and subsequent mental health problems in children. Ed Tronick's mutual regulation model illuminated how Nicole and Haley affected each other in ways that could be helpful or harmful. While I was already familiar with the work of Peter Fonagy, this program allowed me to immerse myself in contemporary research that bridges developmental psychology and neuroscience, showing how the brain grows and develops in relationship with caregivers who respond to the motivations and intentions of children's behavior.

I learned that stress and depression in pregnancy are associated with behavioral dysregulation in babies. Adding to that knowledge is recent evidence that certain medications, such as Prozac, can also have unwanted temporary effects on an infant's behavior. I came to understand Haley and Nicole as a vulnerable mother-baby pair, each bringing qualities to the relationship that were causing a downward spiral of missed cues and miscommunication. I understood how, with those few visits, I offered a holding environment for Haley and her family. It didn't take much time. As this was the time of most rapid brain development, by intervening early I was able to set Haley and the whole family on a healthier path of development.

The Social Womb

The human infant is uniquely helpless in the first weeks and months of life. His arms fly up over his head at random moments in a primitive startle reflex. His sleep patterns have no rhyme or reason. He eats and poops round the clock. This unpredictable behavior is the result of an immature brain that, in the service of human evolution, does 70 percent of its growing outside the womb.

When humans adapted to standing up and walking on two legs, a head that held a fully developed brain could not fit through the narrower birth canal. Also, at nine months' gestation, the metabolic demands of the developing fetus on the mother become too great.

However, in an equally important evolutionary adaptation, the human newborn is available from the earliest hours of life for connection and complex communication. In a calm, quiet setting, at just a few hours of age a baby will turn to his mother's voice, follow her face, and make imitating movements with his mouth. He makes himself available for caregivers to fall in love with him.

These two adaptations come together in the concept of the "social womb," as described by educator and child development researcher J. Ronald Lally. The human infant, with his immaturity but also highly developed capacity for social interaction, "turns this seeming weakness into strength. During this dependent period the human brain is very active, developing more rapidly than at any subsequent period of life."

For the infant to be heard, and so to develop most fully, he needs an environment of caregivers who are available both emotionally and physically, 24 hours a day, seven days a week. For a new human parent, the infant's helplessness may translate to no sleep, no showers, no ability to do anything but care for the baby. This period is sometimes referred to as the fourth trimester, and many books offer advice about how to survive it.

But as Winnicott identified, a mother knows what to do. He referred to this completely consuming kind of care as "primary maternal preoccupation," a preoccupation that is not only healthy but also highly adaptive. Research into the neurobiological and genetic underpinnings of this behavior shows a significant role for oxytocin as well as other neurotransmitters and specific brain structures and neural pathways.

This preoccupation is vital to an infant's development. As Linda Mayes of the Yale Child Study Center summarizes: "In this period, mothers are deeply focused on the infant, to the near exclusion of all else. This preoccupation heightens their ability to anticipate the infant's needs, learn his/her unique signals, and over time to develop a sense of the infant as an individual. Winnicott emphasizes the crucial importance of such a stage for the infant's self-development . . ."

If all goes well, by around three months of age the baby begins to develop the capacity to soothe himself. His movements are no longer random. He can bring his hand to his mouth. His sleep cycles become more regular. A mother can take a shower.

In a beautiful film, *the connected baby*, by developmental psychologist Suzanne Zeedyk, a segment entitled "dance of the nappy" films a mother changing her baby's diaper. The mother speaks in a soft, gentle voice narrating what she is doing and what her baby might be feeling. In this simple and elegant way, Zeedyk shows the exquisite attunement between mother and baby that goes on in countless minute-to-minute interactions throughout the day. It is in this relationship that a baby's brain grows and develops. It is how he develops a sense of himself.

It is only a small step from there to understand that if a mother is, in the words of Winnicott biographer Adam Phillips, "preoccupied with something else," this dance will be significantly altered. When these early months are not protected, when the new family feels unsupported, insecure, or isolated, this time that was anticipated as a period of joy and love may in fact be filled with intense anxiety and loneliness that is all the more painful because it stands in such stark contrast to cultural expectations. Providing the "social womb" the baby's growing brain requires may then be very difficult.

When the expectation exists that a new mother will carry on with her life exactly as she did before the baby was born, with rapid return to her prepregnancy self and body, the attentiveness an infant requires will not only be challenging, it may be impossible. Given the baby's total helplessness—what Winnicott termed "absolute dependence"—in the early weeks and months, this kind of attunement is a full-time job. Not necessarily all done by the mother, but also needing an extended "holding environment" that may include family, friends, and community. As Winnicott wisely observes, "It should be noted that mothers who have it in themselves to provide good-enough care can be enabled to do better by being cared for themselves in a way that acknowledges the essential nature of their task."

There is an evolutionary purpose to what in this country was once termed *lying in*. During a period of three to four weeks, mothers were able to rest and connect with their baby while a group of women helped with household chores and offered emotional support. While modern views of childbirth do not call for prolonged periods of bed rest, this protected time still has great importance. Cultures around the world recognize the need for protecting the mother-baby pair in this way. Contemporary American culture is uniquely lacking in a culture of postpartum care.

A natural consequence of caring for a helpless infant is complete loss of control over one's life. If this is expected, anticipated and accepted as a temporary state, it may pass quickly. Ambivalent feelings about this loss of control, about the complete reorganization of the mother's sense of self, are normal and common, expressed in a beautifully lighthearted fashion by Winnicott:

> Then, one day, they find they have become hostess to a new human being who has decided to take up lodging, and like the character played by Robert Morley in *The Man Who Came to Dinner*, to exercise a crescendo of demands till some date in the far-extended future when there will once again be peace and quiet; and they, these women, may return to self-expression of a more direct kind.

But when mothers don't dare express this ambivalence, when they are alone and increasingly overwhelmed, confused by severe sleep deprivation, normal feelings of ambivalence may become distorted. In a similar way, normal preoccupation may be distorted into intrusive obsessive-compulsive behavior. When, in addition, mothers have increased feelings of self-doubt and low self-esteem, their experience of the transition to parenthood may deteriorate.

Listening to Fathers

Recently I worked with Lauren, a new mom who was struggling terribly with feelings of depression. Her doctor had recommended medication, but she hesitated. Laura's depression lifted when her husband, Tom, started attending a new dads group.

How can we make sense of this? A potential vast disparity exists between a mother's and a father's experience of life with a new infant. A mother usually feels taken care of when her husband takes care of the baby. In contrast, a father, whose spouse may also be *his* sole source of emotional support, may feel alone and abandoned when a mother is—in a natural and healthy way—preoccupied with the baby. At the same time, fathers are often relied upon to be breadwinner, caregiver, as well as primary and sometimes sole source of emotional support for a mother. In addition, many mothers may give mixed signals, asking for help while conveying, in both words and actions, that they know better how to read the baby's signals.

Putting all of these factors together with the helpless infant who requires care 24/7, and both parents may be physically in the same house but feeling terribly alone and disconnected. Depression, for both mother and father, is an understandable result.

In these circumstances, the kind of intense attunement and care the baby demands in these early weeks and months is hard to come by. When his need for preoccupation is not met, a baby may become further disorganized, with an increase in crying along with sleep and feeding difficulties.

A new dads group has the potential to address these issues. Similarly to a moms group, dads can meet others who are having similar struggles. With the baby present, they have the opportunity, in a safe, supportive environment, to learn to read the baby's cues and connect with the baby. When, in turn, a father feels an increased sense of competence, he may become more available both physically and emotionally. A mother may feel less alone and isolated. A positive cycle of connection may be set in place—between mother and father, between parents and baby.

Colic and Primary Maternal Preoccupation

I was recently asked to speak for one hour to a group of medical students as part of their four-week newborn nursery rotation. Challenged to give them a glimpse of the wealth of knowledge I had been exposed to in Tronick's program, I chose to teach them about colic. When you Google *colic*, or ask a range of professionals what it is, you will get responses that places the problem squarely in the baby. By far the most common approach is to first offer parents tips to get the baby to stop crying. When these fail, there may be multiple formula changes and then perhaps a referral to a GI specialist.

But as we saw with Nicole and Haley, the experience of the colicky or fussy baby who cries all the time can be understood only in the context of relationships. I took a completely different approach.

While Winnicott's concept of primary maternal preoccupation is specifically about the early weeks and months when the infant is most helpless, I found a way to illustrate the concept in a work of literature.

The book is James Agee's *A Death in the Family*. In this early scene, the father is awakened during the night because his father is ill. As he dresses to leave the house, his wife, on her way downstairs to make him breakfast, whispers to him to bring his shoes in to the kitchen.

> He watched her disappear, wondering what in hell she meant by that, and was suddenly taken with a snort of silent amusement. She looked so deadly serious, about the shoes. God, the ten thousand little things every day that a woman kept thinking of, on account of children. Hardly even thinking, he thought to himself as he pulled on his other sock. Practically automatic. Like breathing.

I encouraged the students to view colic as a quality in the infant that interferes with this natural process of primary maternal preoccupation. Rather than "breathing," a mother may feel that she is suffocating.

It is hard enough to attend to the needs of a calm, well-regulated newborn. But when that baby startles at the slightest sound, or cries whenever he spits up, or has trouble transitioning from awake to asleep—qualities found in many babies described as "colicky," that primary preoccupation, or what Winnicott termed in his writing for parents, "ordinary devotion," can become extraordinary and even overwhelming. Particularly when a parent feels alone and unsupported, this natural process may be derailed. The relationship may suffer. Qualities in the baby may disrupt this natural give and take between parent and baby. A baby's mood can affect the mother's mood, and a mother's mood can affect the baby's mood. Mother and baby may escalate each other's distress.

With extra help and support, that parent-baby pair can easily get back on track. For Nicole, her own depression and feelings of inadequacy in combination with the severe sleep deprivation turned the "colic" into a growing crisis. I wanted my students to appreciate the value of listening to parent and baby together.

Listening to Postpartum Depression

When I write about postpartum depression, pointing to the social isolation and unrealistic expectations that contribute to the experience, many mothers resonate deeply with this way of thinking. However, a significant number of readers react with the criticism that by bringing in the effects of social and cultural forces, I am implying postpartum depression isn't a "real disease."

Having worked with many new mothers and fathers, I have no doubt that the wide range of serious emotional disturbances that new parents experience are real. Certainly in mothers, hormonal changes that result from pregnancy play a role, though other explanations are in order for fathers, and for the increasingly well-recognized phenomenon of postadoption depression.

I'm suggesting that we understand the forms of emotional distress that occur in the context of caring for a new infant as experiences with complex meaning. Just as we aim to be curious about the meaning of a child's behavior, rather than simply giving his behavior a name, we need to reflect on the meaning of a new parent's experience. Effective treatment of postpartum depression must include opportunity to address the issue in its full social and interpersonal context. This calls for acknowledging the massive biological and psychological shifts of motherhood, the reorganization of the relationship between parents, the role of the baby, as well as the normal ambivalence that accompanies this developmental phase. All this may be distorted in the setting of social isolation, severe sleep deprivation, and unrealistic expectations of rapid return to prepregnancy function.

Calling this experience a disease may be helpful in recognizing the severity of the issue, as well as for getting insurance to cover treatment. Universal postpartum depression screening in the primary care setting, as recently recommended by the US Preventive Services Task Force, will identify mothers whose struggles might otherwise go unrecognized. However, the disease model of biological psychiatry may lead us to try right away to get rid of the symptoms, often with medication alone, without treating the underlying causes. As we saw in Chapter 2, the drug itself can lead to devaluing of listening and neglect of other options. When we place the problem squarely in the mother, without opportunity to explore and understand the social, cultural, and relational context, we are in effect communicating, "There is something wrong with you and I will fix it."

"You have postpartum depression," Cindy's obstetrician told her when she finally developed the courage to speak of her profound emotional pain, her feeling of, as she later told me in my behavioral pediatrics practice, "losing my bearings." He wrote her a prescription for Zoloft and gave her a follow up appointment in a month.

Cindy had struggled with anxiety for years. Now she was alone most of the day with Luke, a fussy baby, while her husband traveled for work. Luke had been diagnosed with food allergies to explain his constant crying, but multiple formula changes failed to improve the situation. Having recently moved, Cindy had few friends in the neighborhood. She described her family of origin as one in which "you didn't talk about feelings." Despite her fragile state of mind and extreme exhaustion, Cindy recognized that while medication could be helpful and even necessary, she did not want only to medicate away her emotional pain.

Somehow, she gathered the strength to find other resources. The first calls she made resulted in offers for appointments in eight to twelve weeks. Through the fog of her distress, she knew this was too late, that she needed an appointment right away, and persevered. She found a therapist who would see her the next week. She told her husband, who while loving and supportive, did not recognize the severity of the situation, that he needed to take some time off to help her. Her pediatrician referred the pair to me. As Cindy felt less alone and in turn more calm, she was able to better help Luke manage his distress, and his crying decreased.

Many new mothers do not have this strength to fight to get help. Offering new parents time and space to be heard, held, and supported is integral to the treatment of postpartum emotional troubles, in both mothers and fathers. This may mean mobilizing family and friends, individual therapy, therapy with parent and infant together, parent-baby groups, or some combination of these. Counseling around sleep, crying, and feeding, as well as yoga, mindfulness, and meditation may also have a role to play, Ideally these supports are available in the earliest months, when not only is the infant most helpless, but also his brain is most rapidly growing.

In my behavioral pediatrics practice, while the fussy baby may be the "identified patient," the mother may be struggling with a range of painful emotional experiences, including depression and anxiety. Working with mother-baby pairs offers an effective way to set development on a healthy path.

"I'm afraid I can't love him," Martha, mother of eight-week-old Benjamin, said to me about fifteen minutes into our first visit. An astute pediatrician had referred Benjamin to me when he was considering admitting the baby to the hospital for "intractable colic." Despite an extensive medical workup, no "cause" had been identified. Still he cried day and night.

In the infant room of my office, a small room with pastel rugs and soft chairs, where on a sunny day the light streamed in through the large window, we had the luxury of an hour in a quiet space to explore her concern. Benjamin was asleep in his car seat for the beginning of this first visit. Martha was able to tell me the following story without interruption. Benjamin had an older brother, Finn, who was "just like this" as an infant. The early years of Finn's life were a traumatic blur for Martha. She herself didn't sleep [very well] for years and remembered it as a time devoid of any joy. Now six years old, Finn had recently been diagnosed with ADHD and there was also a question of whether he might be on the autism spectrum.

Martha described what she termed "post-traumatic stress," as Benjamin seemed to be a similarly fussy and often inconsolable baby. She felt angry all the time and was worried that she might not be able to enjoy her second child.

After a while Benjamin began to fuss. Martha lifted him out of his seat and began to rock him, her agitation visibly increasing as his fussing escalated. Following my hypothesis that this baby, like his older brother, might have some sensory processing challenges (see Chapter 8), I took a rattle that I always have available when evaluating young infants. I gently shook it by his ear. He immediately quieted. When I stopped, the fussing resumed; again he quieted with the rattle. I repeated this three times while Martha watched. We were both convinced that the quiet sound calmed him. Martha was then able to put him down on the blanket where we could continue to talk while observing his behavior.

I noticed that Benjamin intently followed my face. When I began to speak to him while turning my face, at first he continued to follow and to be engaged, but then he got very excited—wildly kicking his arms and legs—and rapidly escalated back to a state of distress. Martha and I observed together how this stimulation could be too much for him, but that he stopped fussing when instead I showed him a red ball. (These tools are all part of the Newborn Behavioral Observation System; see page 49). He even began opening his arms and reaching for it in an immature way. His reaction to my face and voice showed us that he was very interested in people. His tendency to fuss, and to prefer an inanimate object, could be interpreted as an intense response to sensory stimulation, rather than an aversion to social interaction.

The aim of my work was to be present with both Martha and Benjamin, to listen to both at once. Martha began to relax as she in a sense "confessed" her negative feelings about Benjamin. Then she could join me in curiosity about the meaning of Benjamin's be-havior. With space and time for her story to be heard, she naturally shifted her attention to him.

We began to talk about the meaning of our observations. Mar-tha would not be able to protect Benjamin from stimulation, par-ticularly given the high needs of his older brother. But she could begin to make sense of Benjamin's crying from the perspective of how he was experiencing the world. This reinterpreting of his be-havior served to alleviate some of Martha's feelings of helplessness and inadequacy.

We met every three to four weeks over a period of several months. While we observed Benjamin, Martha began to share with me some of the painful experiences she had with her own mother, as well as some of the challenges in her marriage. She was in her own therapy to address these issues, but by bringing them into our work with Benjamin, she could see how her stress affected her in the moment, and work toward separating those feelings from this growing new relationship.

When Benjamin was close to five months, his crying, which had up until that point been subsiding in both amount and inten-sity, suddenly increased. Martha felt a surge of anxiety, express-ing fear that his problems were returning and that all her hard work had been for nothing. But then we did a little experiment. Benjamin was awake and alert when they first arrived. I took him onto my lap, where he had sat comfortably for long periods of time in prior visits. At first he was fine. But he seemed to be study-ing me. Because we were doing nothing else but watching him, we were able to notice that a worried look passed across his face before he broke out into an all-out cry. I handed him back to Martha and immediately he stopped crying. We had clear evidence for a different interpretation, namely that this resurgence in crying represented Benjamin's growing connection with and attachment to his mother. I could point out that this was normal, developmentally appropriate behavior. I also noted that it was a sign of his emerging cognitive skills.

While before this point he certainly knew the difference between his mother and me, he could now think about it in a more sophisticated way. A hectic home setting may lack the opportunity to slow things down in this way. But now that Martha saw the meaning of this resurgence of crying, she not only knew how to manage it, but she could enjoy her baby's new stage of development and attachment to her, rather than falling into overwhelming anxiety.

At this point Martha felt settled and confident. She decided that she and Benjamin no longer needed to see me. About a year later I ran into the pediatrician who had referred the pair to me. He told me that Martha and Benjamin had a "lovely relationship."

Recognizing the Newborn as an Individual

Recognizing the baby as a unique individual with great competencies, while at the same time making sense of vulnerabilities, is the aim of the NBO, or Newborn Behavioral Observation System.

The NBO was developed out of the work of T. Berry Brazelton, the renowned pediatrician and 2012 recipient of President Barack Obama's Presidential Citizens Medal. Winnicott's ideas also reverberate in the NBO. It can be seen as a tool that supports, from the first hours and days of life, a parent's recognition of the child's true self.

Early in his work as a general pediatrician in the 1950s, Brazelton observed the tremendous capacity of the newborn infant for complex communication. In the course of his private practice he saw how a baby, even at a few hours of age, would imitate facial expressions, show rudimentary attempts at reaching, and have different expressions for interactions with an object and with a person's face. Research based on these observations led to development of the Neonatal Behavioral Assessment Scale (NBAS), a way to identify and to evaluate the quality of these newborn capacities. The scale changed the way both child development experts and pediatricians understood babies.

The NBO, developed by psychologist J. Kevin Nugent and colleagues, is a clinical application of the NBAS. It enables a clinician to demonstrate a newborn's unique strengths and vulnerabilities. It can be administered in ten minutes, though in the ideal situation there is more time available to explore feelings that the process inevitably brings up. The NBO literally offers opportunity to make room for this new person in relationship with caregivers and within the family.

Parents who have experienced the NBO often remember it vividly years later. Fathers and siblings can be participants. One study showed a significant decrease in risk for postpartum depression at one month in mothers who experienced the NBO with their infants in the first two days of life. As clinician, I find the occasion is often profound and powerful. Listening to parents and baby together, one is watching the birth of a family.

I use a ninety-second clip of myself doing the NBO with a three-day-old infant and his mother as a teaching tool. The segment is of a section of the NBO referred to as the "orienting items" where the newborn's reaction to an object, face, voice, and voice and face together is observed. At just a few hours of age, many a newborn, much to a parent's delight and amazement, will follow a bright red ball a full 180-degree arc. In this particular segment, we see the baby turn his head to his mother's voice when she speaks softly into his left and then right ear. Although it is not an official part of the NBO, we also see him make rudimentary movements of reach with both arms, overcoming his still strongly present Moro, or startle, reflex. His mother joyfully tells him, "Oh yes, you know me already!" Then I observe his response to my face and voice together. Not only does he follow for two full 180-degree arcs, but he also moves his mouth in sync with my own. I spontaneously say to him, "We're having a real conversation. You're such a little person already."

A Clouded View

While for many parents this recognition of their child's emerging self comes naturally, in the setting of high stress, whether from factors in the parent, the baby, or both, it may not. By taking time to offer the NBO, we make a space for their natural intuition. We encourage the beginning of healthy development of parent and child together. When we identify a newborn's unique traits, we can reframe "problems" as "vulnerabilities." With support, attention, and careful listening, these can be transformed into strengths.

I didn't know it at the time, but my observations alongside Nicole and Dan can be found in the NBAS and NBO. Until we were able to reframe it, Nicole saw her own failure in Haley's "difficult" behavior. Nicole was in a sense projecting her feelings into the behavior she observed in her daughter. She viewed Haley's crying not as a trait in Haley, but as a reflection of her inadequacy.

A parent's own history may color her relationship with her baby, interfering with her ability to see the child as himself. Listening to a parent's story helps to clear away this cloud that is blocking the view. This cloud often takes the form of projection, when a parent puts feelings into a baby that she cannot accept within herself. Projection can take many complex forms. Sometimes, as we will see in Chapter 9, a newborn represents a different person, even from a previous generation.

An ongoing study at Austen Riggs Center, an inpatient psychiatric hospital, is investigating the link, observed in work with patients, between suicidal behavior and a person's belief that he was conceived to fill a role other than himself. By clearing these projections early on, a child is not compelled to play a role.

The story of Marilyn and Steven offers an example. Marilyn's first child, three-year-old Anna, had been an easy baby. Marilyn, who presented herself as a very competent, practical person, could not understand why their second, very fussy infant was unhinging her.

She had been given all sorts of advice and guidance by friends and family. After multiple formula changes, her pediatrician had diagnosed reflux and tried medication. The next step, if things did not improve, was referral to a gastroenterologist. Marilyn felt herself unraveling, and as the weeks went on she was losing her confidence in herself as a mother. She admitted, "Sometimes I think he hates me." She despaired over the loss of the easy intimacy she had shared with Anna before Steven was born. In my office, as she carried her fussing infant, who gradually quieted and fell asleep, she told me the following story.

She was the older of two sisters. For most of her life their relationship had been conflicted and highly troubled (recently she had started therapy to address this very problem). Her sister had been a frail and sickly baby. Marilyn felt that at the age of three, she had been dropped from her parents' mind when the needs of this baby consumed them. She resolved not to repeat this pattern with her own children.

Marilyn paused at this point. With the opportunity to share the story in an unhurried fashion, she seemed to be letting herself experience the pain that was behind her struggles, that she had up until this point blocked out of her mind. Tears filed her eyes and ran down her cheeks as she explained how with the arrival of Steven, she was doing to Anna exactly what her parents had done to her. She admitted to feelings of resentment toward Steven, which were accompanied by overwhelming guilt. She feared that she was not bonded with him.

Now we had a new way to understand her experience of this second baby. While it was true that Steven was a particularly fussy baby, this story offered insight to why Marilyn was becoming unhinged.

With Marilyn's fears out in the open, we could figure out what to do. And clearly it involved more than changing Steven's reflux medication. At that first visit Marilyn was able to share her paralyzing feelings of guilt in a safe and nonjudgmental environment. She was not a "bad" mother for having these conflicted thoughts. We talked about how negative feelings toward a baby are actually quite common and natural. And the difficulties she was facing with a fussy baby were real. As we first began to open up her story, she resisted, insisting that the "problem" lay in Steven alone, that she knew he was a baby who cried more than normal. But when over time she connected with the deeper painful feelings, and was given permission to grieve openly in my office, there was a sense of relief in the room. The guilt and anger that had been in the way of connecting with her new baby dissipated.

The "problem" was that Marilyn needed to find a way to love both children comfortably at the same time. I suggested that I meet with the whole family together. By having both children in the room, Marilyn could talk with me about what she was experiencing in real time. We could brainstorm about how to find time for closeness with each child alone, given her husband's busy work schedule.

One reward for this work was a blossoming relationship between Steven and Anna. As Marilyn increasingly found her own center and was able to be more present for both children, she saw Anna begin to enjoy her big sister role. In one particularly delightful moment, Anna repeatedly held the toy stethoscope in my office to her baby brother's chest as both children dissolved in laughter.

Steven was indeed a very fussy baby, and central to the treatment was both validation of Marilyn's experience, and concrete support and guidance for managing this behavior. But equally important was learning the meaning of his behavior for Marilyn. In a sense my role was as interpreter, helping Marilyn to separate her own meaning from the meaning for Steven.

We could observe his rhythms and his sensory processing sensitivities. Marilyn noticed that sometimes after carrying him for hours trying to make him stop crying, he was calm the moment she put him down. In a classic example of projection, Anna had been placing her own intolerable feelings onto Steven. It was she who was rejecting him because his needs interfered in her relationship with her daughter. But because this was an intolerable feeling, she had projected her feelings onto him, insisting that his behavior represented a rejection of her.

But now Marilyn could see Steven's actual needs. Unlike Anna, who had been a very cuddly infant, Steven seemed to feel calmer when he observed the world on his own. This was a side of Steven's nature that she could understand and respect. She began to recognize his true self.

In my practice I am able to listen to parent and baby together, observing how interactions lead to either distress or connection. We can pay attention to the way a baby affects a parent and parent affects a baby. When the issues are deep and complex, as in the case of Steven and his mother, this protected time can be essential to setting development on a healthy path.

Obstacles to Investing in Infants

Research of Pulitzer Prize–winning economist James Heckman is frequently cited as evidence supporting the need for investment in early childhood. Recently, much of this discussion has focused on preschool for all, starting at age four. However, all the best science of our time tells us that investing in early childhood means investing in infancy. This is when our "return on investment" is the greatest, because the brain is most rapidly growing and changing. Neuroplasticity, or ability to change the brain, occurs throughout life. But when we listen while the brain is actively growing and changing, we have the opportunity for primary prevention. It takes much less time to set a family on a different path when we take the time early on to address the ways in which development is being derailed.

Psychoanalysts for over a hundred years have recognized the significance of early relationships in health and development. Now the exploding science of early childhood offers evidence that early parental care regulates physiology, influences development of a healthy stress response, and affects the expression of genes and structure and function of the brain.

But the science may not benefit families if our culture does not value parents in the way the research suggests is critically important. For many countries, having a home visitor to support new parents in the early weeks and months is standard. In Finland, every new parent receives a "baby box" filled with clothes, diapers, and other assorted baby needs. When the box is empty, it often serves as the baby's first bed. While the items themselves are useful, the meaning of this box is of great significance. It says, "Our society places value on new parents and babies."

In contrast, our country has one of the most restrictive parental leave policies in the world; it is one of only two developed countries that do not have government-supported paid maternity leave. With this lack of investment in parents and infants, many families may find it impossible to offer the care that research shows is needed in the early weeks, months, and years.

Beatrice Beebe, a leading researcher in infant development whose detailed videotapes of mothers and infants offer elegant evidence for the richness and complexity of early parent-child relationships, suggested to a pediatrician colleague that video be used in every four-month well child visit. Replaying of videotape, when parents, together with a clinician, can watch themselves interacting with their infant, has been shown to be a useful clinical tool in promoting healthy relationships. The science certainly supports such investment in time and attention to parent-child relationships in infancy. But in today's fast-paced world of primary care, where clinicians are under pressure to see more and more patients in less and less time, such a suggestion is almost laughable.

Four

Listening as Prevention

It is easier to build strong children than to repair broken men.

—*Frederick Douglass*

As we have seen in the last chapter, listening to infant and parents is a powerful first step to preventing mental health problems and troubled relationships later in childhood. Steve and Deb Boczenowski, two brave, thoughtful, and kind people, founded TADS (Teenage Anxiety and Depression Solutions) in the wake of their son Jeffrey's suicide at the age of twenty-one. Steve and Deb work tirelessly to ensure that other families do not suffer lost and alone, as they did in the face of their son's declining mental health. Recently Steve invited me to speak to an audience of preschool parents and teachers. In his introduction he explained that while this might seem an unlikely audience for such an organization, he recognized how early signs of difficulty may be present in elementary school and even before. He wanted parents to know that they should not struggle by themselves, but should get help.

I spoke to this audience about listening to a child's communication and giving space and time to grow into her true self. At the
end of my talk, a mother raised her hand. She began to speak tearfully about her five-year-old son who became overwhelmed with
anxiety in multiple settings—going to school, birthday parties, or
swim lessons. She wondered whether she shouldn't get help, rather
than simply listen.

I took great care to correct this misconception, as the whole
point of the event was exactly the opposite, namely that when a
young child and family are struggling, that is the time to get help.
It is a question of what kind of help. I wanted her to feel understood and supported, as she clearly was in great pain over her son's
struggles. I encouraged her to find help from a person—be it her
pediatrician or some kind of therapist (as we will see in Chapter 8,
an occupational therapist who works with a child's sensory sensitivities can be a great resource) who would listen to her story and
support her efforts to make sense of her son's behavior and think
creatively about how to help him manage his particular sensitivities. Sometimes I will take an entire hour-long session to talk about
one such incident at a swim lesson or birthday party, so as to understand the full complexity of the experience for both parent and
child. I cautioned this mother against what may at first seem the
easier path of finding out "what was wrong with him." I wanted to
call attention to the important distinction between *managing* and
understanding.

We are learning more every day about how this early life experience of being understood leads to a child's ability to regulate
her emotions. In other words, when parents let a child know that
a birthday party can be difficult for her, and that together they
can make sense of it, this understanding presence is in the long
run of more value than whether they choose on any given day to

stick it out or go home. Many parents fret over what to do in such a situation, when in fact each choice has its pluses and minuses. However, having a parent who gets what is going on for her will help a child to have a better sense of herself, and so increase her ability to handle similar situations in the future.

Compelling Evidence from Adults

A large long-term study sponsored by the CDC (Centers for Disease Control) whose far-reaching implications are increasingly being recognized, offers dramatic evidence of the value of listening to children and families as primary prevention. The Adverse Childhood Experiences (ACE) Study has its origins in exploration of the causes of adult obesity. Researchers were surprised to find that the greatest predictors of adult obesity were painful or traumatic childhood experiences. Decades of research have now shown that these experiences—not only abuse and neglect, but also the more ubiquitous experiences of such things as parental mental illness, substance abuse, domestic violence, and divorce—are additive. The greater number of these experiences, or the higher the ACE score, the more likely a person is to have a range of significant health problems, both physical and mental. These early experiences get under our skin, into our body and brain. This study has implications, as I discuss in Chapter 6, for how we treat older children and adults with a range of health concerns. But perhaps most important, the ACE study shows that we need to devote resources to early childhood. We need to listen for the story of the parent who struggles with depression or alcoholism, or who loses her cool and grabs her child and shakes him. We need to help parents whose marriage is faltering not to feel shame, but rather to get help. But when the child's efforts to communicate distress in the face of these and similar experiences is instead labeled as a disorder, "managed" and/or medicated, not only is the child's communication silenced, but we also lose the opportunity to address these issues early and prevent them from exerting their harmful effects.

Listening Changes the Brain

An explosion of research at the interface of developmental psychology, genetics, and neuroscience shows us that this approach of finding meaning in a child's behavior affects not only that behavior but also the structure and biochemistry of the brain. This research offers evidence that early experience influences gene expression and thus the way the brain develops. Termed *epigenetics*—literally "above the gene"—this rapidly expanding field of study focuses not on the sequence of DNA in our genes, that is fixed and unchanging, but rather the regulation of activity of those genes. In a fascinating review of this complex field of study, Columbia University researchers explain that the quality of parent-child interactions produce epigenetic changes in the brain that account for variation in stress response, thinking capacities, and social competence.

This does not mean that the lack of listening and understanding at a particular time in childhood dooms a child's development. The study of epigenetics, and our growing knowledge about the plasticity of the brain, gives us reason to believe that even when a child's development goes off track when there are significant disruptions, there is opportunity for growth and change throughout life. However, with the rapid development of the brain in the earliest weeks, months, and years, we have the opportunity to set development on a healthy path from the start.

This kind of early prevention works in many settings. John Green and colleagues at the University of Manchester have shown how listening to parent and child together can set a child at risk for autism on a different path. His group studied infants with an older sibling with a diagnosis of autism. These infants have a twenty-fold increase in risk of receiving the diagnosis. In one randomly assigned group, a therapist sat on the floor with a parent and child and supported the parent in making sense of the child's communication. While the study is ongoing, the first round of published results at fourteen-month follow-up showed children receiving this form of intervention displaying fewer autistic-like behaviors than the group who did not receive this supportive treatment.

While this study is specifically about autism, it has relevance for any parent-infant pair that is having trouble trying to connect. This difficulty may stem from issues in the parent, as with postpartum depression, the child, as when her signals are difficult to read, or both. A person who has a relationship with the parent, who offers space and time to listen to parent and child together, makes all the difference.

Given what we know about the plasticity of the brain, rather than framing the question as "Does a young child have a disorder or not?" we might ask instead, "How do we hold parents through a period of uncertainty (a concept I elaborate on in Chapter 10) to give a child the best opportunity to grow into her true self? As Green's research beautifully demonstrates, patience during a period of uncertainty does not translate to "do nothing."

Holding in Groups

Mother-baby groups—and father-baby groups—also can create a safe, containing, holding environment, supporting parent and baby together. Such groups offer an enormous opportunity for promoting healthy development. When parents feel held by the group, they have more energy to hold their baby, both physically and emotionally.

I had the privilege of watching this strengthening bond develop as a consultant to the eight-week new mothers groups, with the lovely title "Balance After Baby," offered as a community service by the Freedman Center at William James College in Newton, Massachusetts. I observed how, when an effective leader sets a warm, nonjudgmental tone, at the first session mothers often share feelings of sadness, anxiety, and loneliness. Over the eight-week period I witnessed significant transformations, as mothers gained confidence and deep, intimate knowledge of their babies. Well-run groups can create a time of remarkable growth and healing.

When I attend the group, my title of "MD" incurs the risk that I am identified as the "expert," and so parents ask me what to do about a range of problems. One mom, Sharon, asked about her four-month-old infant, "What books should I read to know how to start solids?"

She had asked her pediatrician this same question multiple times, but as of yet none of the answers she received had satisfied her. She was looking for something that she had so far not been able to express. So, rather than directly answering her question again, I observed that it seemed hard for her to imagine how her baby would communicate her needs. Only then did we learn the full story. She began telling the group about how feeding her daughter was so filled with stress that she could not enjoy it. She then shared with us her experiences that were in the way of her recognizing that her daughter would naturally go from nursing every two hours to eating three meals a day with the family.

Alison had been only 5 pounds at birth. "How will I know that I'm giving her enough?" Sharon asked. Her voice cracked, and tears began to flow. Her question about starting solids was linked to this deep, yet until now unexpressed, fear about Alison's physical vulnerability. "But," she said hesitantly, "I know she's a healthy, vigorous baby." Sharon was looking for a validation of her natural intuition.

As she went on, filling the open space that the group offered, she shared her deeper concern—her husband's anxiety. His worry over the baby's size was even greater than hers. She feared that he would question her, shaking her tenuous confidence in Alison's health. This issue in her marriage, along with anxiety stemming from the baby's low birth weight, was interfering with her finding her way as a mother. She and her husband were navigating their new roles of being parents together and needed to find ways to support, not undermine, each other.

With the story out in the open, Sharon became more able to connect with her natural intuition, and feeding her baby became a source of pleasure. One of the other moms in the group wisely observed how our culture of advice, with the explosion of material in books and on the Internet, could all serve to undermine a parent's natural intuition.

A recent article in the journal *Pediatrics* titled "Teaching the Essentials of "Well Child Care" addresses this issue, calling for pediatricians to ask "open-ended questions," followed by "anticipatory guidance." Anticipatory guidance, a term introduced by T. Berry Brazelton in 1975 and incorporated into his Touch-points theory and programs, offers a way to point out the next developmental landmarks, with their inherent disruptions, and prevent possible troubles. But, as I will explore in the following chapter, with current pressures to see more and more patients in less and less time, what may be lacking in this scenario is time for open-ended answers.

One might imagine that had Sharon not had an opportunity to voice her true concerns, her worries about her baby's eating habits might have become magnified. Often parental anxieties about a baby's physical vulnerability are at the root of later distorted relationships around food and eating. Her pediatrician had answered her question with standard nutritional advice. But the advice fell on deaf ears since the underlying reason for the question went unaddressed. While her pediatrician repeatedly told her what percentile the baby was on, Sharon told the group, echoing Winnicott's concept of the true self, "I don't want her to be a percentile—I want her to be a person!"

The Emerging Self: Listening to Toddlers

When calling attention to the value of investment of resources in the early years of childhood, many refer to the rapid brain development when trillions of brain cell connections are made. While the phrase "trillions of brain cells" feels abstract, just spend time with a toddler, where the explosion of thinking, language, and motor skills accompanies the emergence of a distinctive person, and this "science" will become very real. In a recent article about the first year of life, writer Yudhijit Bhattacharjee beautifully juxtaposes brain science with the wonder of child development:

> If the metamorphosis of a cluster of cells into a suckling baby is one of life's great miracles, so is the transformation of that wobbly infant into a walking, talking toddler capable of negotiating bedtime. While researching this story, I have watched that miracle unfold before my eyes as my daughter has gone from a fidgety bundle with only a piercing cry signaling hunger to a feisty three-year-old who insists on putting on her sunglasses before stepping out of the house.

Listening to toddlers and their parents makes it possible to appreciate the wonder of this transformation. Just as in our culture parents may not be allowed time to adjust to and enjoy the birth of a newborn, parents may not have the opportunity to reflect on this major developmental shift (particularly when it coincides, as it does in many families, with the arrival of a newborn).

Instead of being seen as the exciting emergence of a new more complex self, toddlerhood has been branded as the "terrible twos." The rather sudden presence of an individual who can say no may unsettle the family dynamic, but taking time to pay attention can help repair these natural disruptions. In a busy household, however, a negative pattern of interaction may insidiously take hold. Noah's story is one example.

Unlike many of the young children I see in my practice, three-year-old Noah was described by his parents, Adam and Janet, as an easy, "delightful" baby. When he turned two, however, shortly before the birth of his brother, they began to notice what they called "defiant" behavior. They described a household filled with conflict and anger. Now he was constantly in time-out, and showing ever-increasing aggression toward his baby brother. His pediatrician referred the family to me after a couple of incidents of shoving other kids in his new preschool. They were concerned he might be "kicked out."

For the first thirty minutes of our visit, Janet and Adam spoke about Noah in quite negative terms—"controlling," "defiant," "stubborn," and the ambiguous, but usually negatively tinged "strong-willed." But as they began to relax, in the expanse of time and quiet before us, deep feelings of sadness emerged. Janet spoke sadly of longing to reconnect with her son in a loving way and to be free of the anger that seemed to now fill their days. As they were leaving, almost as an afterthought, she mentioned the difficult delivery of her second child, Will.

When I met with the family the following week, while Noah played with the array of toys, I opened up this subject again. The rage that was gripping Janet seemed to have loosened. She spoke of "letting things go" and not going head to head with him about everything. Already the mood in the house had shifted subtly. But when she again had the opportunity to vent her frustrations, she began to tell me how "difficult" Noah had been on a recent outing. At this point, Noah, who had been playing calmly, began to bang a toy on the metal cabinet, disrupting our conversation. I noticed together with Janet and Adam that he was clearly taking in what we were saying, reacting to the negative language. Perhaps this was a good time to explore the story of the birth of his brother, both to divert this negative attention, and gain further insight to how things had become derailed.

It was the Fourth of July at a big family gathering, a month before her due date. Janet had suddenly felt ill, and she and Adam left the party for the hospital, leaving Noah with his grandparents. Janet had severe preeclampsia and that night Will was delivered by emergency C-section. Janet had been intubated in the ICU for several days after the birth. Will was in the special care nursery with a number of complications. Both mother and baby recovered. But Will was a very fussy newborn who cried all the time and never slept.

As Janet told this story approaching Will's first birthday, Janet and Adam allowed themselves really to feel their fear for the first time. Janet reflected that she was "glad they were both alive." In the blur of caring for a toddler and this high-needs infant, neither she nor Adam had the chance to reflect on this major disruption in their lives, to consider its effect on them and on Noah. Janet told me that she had not even had a chance to prepare Noah, and recognized that seeing her in the ICU where, she gently acknowledged, "I really didn't look good," might have been frightening for him.

We now had the chance to reframe his "defiant" behavior. Just at the time when children learn to name and control their big toddler feelings, his parents were preoccupied and highly stressed. I suggested that we think of the problem developmentally, and recognize that because of these events, perhaps Noah was a bit behind in his ability to manage his emotions. When he got upset, as at that recent outing where he began to lash out, he needed both support and limits on his behavior, as if he were a younger child. His advanced verbal skills made it difficult for his parents to see this emotional immaturity.

As the time to leave the office approached, we could see that Noah was going to offer us an example of his "defiance." When his parents told him it was time to clean up and leave, he asked for a snack. They both said no, and that he could have it in the car. He then stuck in his heels and refused to help. The tension in the room rapidly escalated.

I took advantage of the opportunity to listen and reframe in real time. "Perhaps this leaving is stressful for him and having a snack will help him feel calm." "But," Adam asked, "won't that mean I'm giving in to his manipulative behavior?" Again I tried to present the situation from a different angle. Adam was still in charge. He was making the decision to help Noah with the transition while avoiding a meltdown.

When I met with Janet a few weeks later, she described a significant transformation with "75 percent less trouble" and an emerging loving relationship between Noah and his brother. These few hours together, with space and time to listen to the story, offered this family an opportunity to hit the reset button and take a different path. While we are not able to see the "trillions of brain cell connections," when we observe the dramatic shifts in behavior and relationships that listening promotes, we know that it is doing its work of changing the brain.

Listening over Time

These stories of reframing behavior and vivid improvement are not meant to imply that a few sessions of listening will solve all problems or permanently repair relationships. But by working in this very focal way, to help parent and child connect in the moment, the relationship and the child's development can be set on a different trajectory. Inevitably new concerns will arise, whether from stressful life events, the child's developmental strides, or both. The very nature of development calls for this kind of listening over time.

Janet called me about a year after this visit concerned about a resurgence of Noah's aggressive behavior. He was doing well in school, making friends and learning with no further incidents of aggression. When we met again, already some of Janet's initial panic had abated as she realized that her worries that he would be kicked out of school had been unfounded. She saw how the changes that had occurred in the wake of our meetings seemed, at least in part, to have been long lasting.

With a full-hour visit ahead of us, she began by telling me about her current pregnancy and the need to buy a bigger house. They had just put their home on the market. Uncertainty about the changes, in particular about the likely need to put Noah in a different school, had created a lot of stress at home. She and Adam had fallen into old habits, finding it easy to direct anger and frustration at Noah, who was the more likely of the two children to respond to stress with inflexibility. His newly forming skills of emotional regulation could easily go "off-line."

This kind of regression is a well-recognized problem. Psychiatrist Bruce Perry has developed a model of treatment, the Neurosequential Model of Therapeutics, based on the observation that when children have experienced disruptions in development, under stress they may revert to functioning at the level of development they had reached at the time of the original problem. When this happens, addressing the problem in sequence, by interacting with the child as if he were still at that earlier stage, offers the best chance for return to more age-appropriate behavior.

With this opportunity to regroup, Janet and Adam found their way back to setting limits while at the same time offering support. They stopped trying to reason with him in the middle of a meltdown, and instead, thinking back to how effective this approach had been the first time we met, conveyed love and reassurance. Our initial work together had given them a model for this kind of interaction, and it did not take long for the family to reset and get back on a smoother path.

The problem between Noah and his parents recurred in the face of stressful life events. Paula and Ian's story offers an example of how new concerns may arise, not only because of an external event, but also in the face of a new stage of development. I initially worked with Paula and her infant son Ian shortly after her hospitalization for severe postpartum depression. I helped them find their way following this significant disruption, and they did well. In fact, when Paula called me a few years later with the concern that Ian "wouldn't listen," she told me that the past two years had been "the best years of my life." But now there were daily battles about everything, especially when getting ready to leave for school and at bedtime.

As we spoke at our first visit, alone without Ian, Paula shared persistent debilitating feelings of guilt over what she thought of as her "abandonment" of him when he was an infant. She told me, "I left him once, and I'll never do it again." But now, the time had come when it was developmentally appropriate for Ian to leave *her*. She was anticipating his every need, not letting him experience any frustration. But by making herself so completely available to him, in a sense being the "too good mother," she was getting in his way. She needed to feel comfortable letting him go, and to convey to him that it was okay for him to separate from her. While he might at first resist bedtime or drop off at preschool, she needed to confidently set limits, rather than acquiesce when he resisted. Once we had given words to these feelings, she found his behavior around moments of separation, both leaving for school and going to sleep, to be significantly less fraught.

At each step in the journey of parenting, patient and sensitive listening continues to be needed. New issues inevitably arise, and worries that there is "something wrong" with a child keep cropping up. Labels and quick fixes continue to be tempting.

But when parents experience early on the transformative effects of listening carefully, then when new concerns arise, rather than asking, "How do I manage this behavior?" the stage is set to search for understanding, in turn getting development back on track.

A conversation I had with Evan's mother, Claire, toward the end of his second year of college offers an example of this phenomenon at the other end of the developmental spectrum. Evan had had a recurrence of his anxiety midway through the year. Claire would answer his distraught texts right away, and found herself increasingly embroiled in difficult conversations that rapidly trended downward. Sensing this unhealthy pattern, she went for a consultation with her own therapist. She told me that in their work she realized that her immediate response to his distress came from a fear that he would feel forgotten—a fear that arose from her own childhood experience. "He doesn't feel that way," she understood in an "aha" moment. "The fear is mine," she said, "not his." This insight led her to wait an hour at a minimum before responding to Evan's texts. Both she and her son were pleased to discover that with this approach Evan was well able to shift himself out of these helpless and disorganized states. Now, she told me, he was preparing for a semester abroad, something neither of them could have imagined him doing a year earlier.

As we learn to value listening in relationships, starting with babies offers the best chance for prevention. But no matter at what age, listening is effective only if we have adequate space and time. The common "I don't have time for myself," heard from a parent, as well as the statements from professionals that they are not supported adequately for time spent listening, are not idle complaints, but rather the essence of the problem. The following chapter will explain why the actual numbers of minutes, as well as the physical space, are essential to listening that promotes healing, growth, and resilience.

Five

Time and Space for Listening

In his book *The Examined Life*, psychoanalyst Stephen Grosz offers a beautiful example of the link between time and listening. In considering the effects of excess meaningless praise on children, he describes observing an experienced teacher:

> I watched Charlotte with a four-year-old boy, who was drawing. When he stopped and looked at her—perhaps expecting praise—she smiled and said, "There's a lot of blue in your picture." He replied, "It's the pond near my grandmother's house—there is a bridge." He picked up a brown crayon, and said, "I'll show you." Unhurried, she talked to the child, but more importantly she observed, she listened. She was present.

In today's fast-paced world, we often feel pressed for time. When parents of young children work long hours and come home exhausted at the end of the day, the idea of "quality time" is elusive. We wonder why meltdowns always occur just when we are trying to get dinner ready. When we slow things down, taking time to make sense of this behavior, it becomes clear that a child, in need of this kind of full presence, is asking a parent, "Just be with me." A meltdown at that inopportune time may be a consequence of the strain of holding it together all day, and now feeling the safety to fall apart. But a parent who is herself exhausted may interpret this end of the day tantrum as willfully "making my life difficult." To slow down, or even stop, and listen may feel impossible in the face of anger and frustration. One mother, given an opportunity in conversation with me to notice an unhelpful pattern, made a beautiful adaptation to this dilemma. After she had spent a long, difficult day dealing with dysfunctional office dynamics, her three-year-old daughter's demands for imaginary play overwhelmed her already taxed brain. But she discovered that coloring together, with her daughter sitting on her lap, offered them a chance to connect while at the same time engaging in an activity that was calming for both.

In her book *Overwhelmed: Work, Love, and Play When No One Has the Time*, author Brigid Schulte points to the fact that in contrast to Denmark, where leisure time without children is valued and protected, American mothers, on average, have about thirty-six minutes a day to themselves. My yoga teacher spent a year teaching in Israel where childcare was offered during most of their classes, and, in her words, "The mothers' right to take care of themselves so that they could take care of their families was encouraged and supported."

In her own studio, modeled on what she experienced in Israel, this teacher takes a few minutes at the beginning of each yoga class to share thoughts, offering a theme for the class, and reflecting how many experiences of life are "just like in yoga." That time at the beginning to settle in helps us be fully present in the practice. The space in which I wrote much of this book, a small coffee shop in Great Barrington with a regular cast of characters, with the quiet background hum of conversation, when I had an expanse of time to work, offered a peaceful calm. As in yoga, it took some time to settle in, some rambling, and some words that eventually got deleted, before I found my way to what I really meant to communicate.

One young mother, pregnant with her third child, wanted to know what was "wrong" with her three-year-old son who "didn't listen." She herself had recently been diagnosed with ADHD. Rather than recognize that her distractibility was due in large part to chronic sleep deprivation along with having too much to keep track of with no support, she was diagnosed with a disorder. She acknowledged frequently yelling at her son and "losing her cool." We discovered that lack of both time and space was at the root of their struggles. Her husband had a new job that required both long hours and a long commute. Not only did she not have time to care for herself, but also, as their house was undergoing major renovations, she and her children had no safe place in which to play. My initial approach to treatment of her son's "behavior problem" focused on helping her create that safe space in her home and carve out some time for going to the gym, an activity that she found calming and that had previously been a major part of her life. When finding time for self-care seems unattainable, it may increase pressure to locate the problem in the child.

While the lack of time and space is ubiquitous in our culture, and the need to protect both relevant to all aspects of our lives, this chapter will focus on how it affects the setting in which a child is being evaluated and treated for "problem behavior." The lack of opportunity for calm reflection in this setting is inextricably linked with the current explosion of psychiatric diagnosis and treatment.

Drawing on his experience as a psychoanalyst, Winnicott described the importance of the setting in his work with adult patients. The reliability of the appointment time, the quiet and comfort of the room, the way the clinician is fully present with the patient, all have an important role to play. A number of years ago I had the good fortune to have a therapist who was heavily influenced by Winnicott. Now, long after I have stopped seeing him, when I run into a difficult situation, with work, family, or other stressors, and find myself becoming unhinged, I pause for a moment. I take a deep breath, and in my mind I bring myself back to his office. The words exchanged had been important, but simply being in his presence, in that quiet, comfortable place, was calming and regulating. The whole experience was central to the treatment, and I can make use of it years later.

The time needed is not limitless. In fact, in psychotherapy, the end of the session is equally as important as the beginning. We need to be able to engage in the world, whether as a child, parent, or professional, while also having a time when we feel held, heard, and recognized. For Evan in Chapter 2, his parents listened to him on the phone, but they encouraged him to stick it out, to give life a chance to be the "treatment" he needed. His work and his relationships at school were eventually what helped him make that necessary separation. While he knew his parents were there for him, he found new opportunities for holding environments in his adult life.

Similarly when a child's development gets off track, by taking the time to listen, rather than jump to give advice, professionals who care for children can support parents in reconnecting with their own natural expertise. While I convey to families who are struggling that I am available, and should new issues emerge they can always come back, we are working together toward a time when parents can say with confidence, "We've got this."

Time to Feel Safe

Connection and social engagement are hard to come by when we don't feel safe. When parents come to my office a cool and collected external appearance may belie a state of intense stress, fear, and even shame that inevitably accompany the question "Is there something wrong with my child?" The very act of taking a history can feel threatening. I notice that the first part of a meeting with parents, even if I have met them before, has a completely different feel and tone from the second. With an expanse of time before us to let the story unfold, while accepting the full range of their feelings without judgment, the sense of threat will subside.

I am struck again and again by the ease with which the story usually emerges. I have wondered whether in part this is due to my title of "pediatrician" rather than "mental health professional." In an age where significant stigma around mental illness still exists, the act of seeking help for a child from a psychotherapist or psychiatrist may be particularly threatening, leading parents to be more guarded than they are with me. It may take longer to feel safe.

When a number of years ago I shifted from my general pediatric practice to focus exclusively on behavioral pediatrics, the only thing that changed was the length of the visits, which went from fifteen minutes to a full hour. But that simple change brought dramatic results. A family and I could settle into our work. Often, once parents had time to escape from the frenetic pace of life, and could talk and be heard, the change in their demeanor would be dramatic as they went from tense and angry to soft, calm, or even sad. I found myself literally taking a deep breath, bringing myself into the moment. Children went from chaotic exploration to calm, engaged play. Sometimes a child would respond to his parent's changed tone by spontaneously running to give him or her a hug. In these powerful moments of reconnection I would feel a tingling in my arms and tears in my eyes. By using our time together not for behavior management, parent training, or parent education, but simply to listen, transformations, for the parent and child, and for me, occurred in our body and brain.

Parents may feel deeply threatened by a child's behavior. A meltdown in public may lead to intense feelings of shame. Or on a still deeper level, if, for example, a parent has as a child experienced abuse, when a toddler loses control and hits, he may provoke a reaction out of proportion to his behavior, leading that parent to shut down. A similar kind of shutting down can occur when a parent seeks professional help for a child who is struggling.

What happens in our body and brain in these situations that makes it impossible to connect? Research by Stephen Porges, a neuroscientist at University of North Carolina, offers an understanding of the biology of both. Porges refers to the way we assess the safety of a situation as "neuroception." Prior to Porges's discovery, there were thought to be two ways in which our nervous system can function during interaction with our environment. When we feel safe, the parasympathetic system is active and we are calm and engaged. The sympathetic system, that controls the well-known fight-or-flight response, becomes active in the face of threat or fear. Porges identified a third way that our nervous system reacts, also under control of the parasympathetic system. This response takes over in the face of overwhelming threat, leading us to shut down. Two different branches of the vagus nerve, which makes up the parasympathetic system, control engagement and shutting down, with the more moderated response of the sympathetic system sandwiched in between. He terms this finding the "polyvagal theory." The branch he calls the "smart vagus" is active when we are open to receive a hug, to look into a person's eyes, to listen and connect. In a second stage of response, when we sense danger, the sympathetic fight-or-flight response kicks in. The third stage is controlled by the branch of the parasympathetic system he calls the "primitive vagus." This branch, active in the "freeze response" that leads an animal to play dead, takes over in the face of overwhelming threat.

This discovery has particular relevance for parents. They may feel threatened both by their child's behavior and in the doctor's office, but the natural drive to protect their child makes either fight or flight impossible, and so may override the sympathetic response. The more primitive stress response takes over. Under the influence of the primitive vagus, even the muscles of the ear do not work properly, literally interfering with the ability to listen. The facial muscles, identified by Darwin as central to expression of emotion, respond differently to the primitive vagus. Frozen facial muscles are an outward expression of what is commonly termed dissociation.

Porges's polyvagal theory helps explain why taking time for nonjudgmental listening in a safe, containing space can be healing for parent and child alike. In his introduction to Porges's book, psychiatrist and trauma researcher Bessel Van der Kolk writes: "Porges . . . gave us an explanation why a kind face and a soothing tone of voice can dramatically alter the entire organization of the human organism—that is, how being seen and understood can help shift people out of disorganized and fearful states." In that first half-hour of a visit, when parents settle in and begin to feel safe, the feeling of threat subsides, and so the smart vagus can come back on line. Connection becomes possible.

The Play Space

Winnicott identified his office and appointments as a kind of play space. "It is in playing and only in playing that the individual child or adult is able to be creative and to use the whole personality, and it is only in being creative that the individual discovers the self."

Later in the same work, he points to the role of space and time in healing. Therapy, in his view, must "afford opportunity for formless experience, and for creative impulses, motor and sensory, which are the stuff of playing." When Winnicott refers to "playing," he does not mean "play therapy" but the opportunity—literally in the case of a child, and more figuratively with an adult—to sit on the floor and see what happens.

Dancing Lessons, a play premiered at Barrington Stage Company in 2014, ostensibly about an actual dancing lesson, offers an example. An injured dancer reluctantly agrees to give a one-hour dance lesson to a young man with Asperger's syndrome who lives in her apartment building.

At first the two characters are cast in conventional roles, he awkwardly defining himself by listing *DSM* diagnostic criteria for autism, and she drinking too much while spewing bitterness over her unexpected disability. Over the course of the play's single act, as their relationship deepens, we appreciate the complexity of their characters. As they grow closer, sharing painful stories of loss from their past, they discover they are in many ways not that different from each other. In a wonderful fantasy sequence at the end, the two shed their respective disabilities and dance gracefully together, playing and healing.

As we have seen, parent-child relationships can be a complex, intricate dance. At times this dance can be full of mismatches and stepped-on toes. Sitting on the floor and playing, with a therapist who is listening to parent and child together, can be a form of dancing lessons. Feeling safe and free, parent and child learn to dance gracefully and to find joy in their relationship.

Highlighting this connection between creativity and mental health, every summer the Austen Riggs Center in Stockbridge, Massachusetts, hosts a creativity seminar in which mental health clinicians and a range of artists come together to explore the creative process. In the introduction to *A Spirit That Impels*, a collection of essays that grew out of the yearly seminar, editor M. Gerard Fromm shares a vignette told to him by a colleague who had the good fortune to observe Winnicott at work. This particular consultation involved a young mother and her three-year-old son.

"He sat on the floor playing with the child, while also talking with the mother, who was sitting on the couch. She told Winnicott that her ordinarily sweet little boy had suddenly become quite ill-tempered and obstreperous. Worst of all, toilet training was completely set back, and the lad was now worrisomely constipated. The father in this working-class household spent long hours at two jobs, and the boy's mother was at her wit's end."

Fromm's colleague described how she had no idea what was going on, but at the end of the visit Winnicott turned to the mother and said, "So, how long have you been pregnant?" Startled by the question, his mother replied that she had not told anyone, but Winnicott thought that the boy did in fact know and suggested she speak with him about it. When the mother returned a few weeks later, she reported that not only was her son "great fun again," but his constipation had completely resolved.

This playfulness that Winnicott employed in his clinical work stands in stark contrast to today's system of mental health care replete with assessment tools and standardized forms. A structured set of questions restricts the possible answers. It is the very lack of structure, essential to play, that leads to understanding and meaningful solutions.

My work is not play therapy, in which play is used to help a child express his thoughts and feelings. Rather, in a way that I hope is similar to Winnicott, I aim to introduce a kind of playfulness to the evaluation. By suggesting that we sit on the floor and see what happens—the child may not even play—it frees us all to let the situation unfold. I do not know how Winnicott figured out from the visit that this boy's mother was pregnant. But clearly his stool holding was connected to that "withheld" piece of information. When I can manage my own as well as a parent's anxiety about the lack of structure, similar insights emerge.

Eliza's parents came to me overwhelmed by concern over their daughter's "shy" behavior. They had a hard time tolerating her lack of communication in the office, repeatedly pushing her to talk to me. Upon learning that their daughter loved to sing, I asked whether she would sing something for me. She wouldn't say a word, but with her back to me, initially almost inaudibly but then with growing confidence, sang an entire song. She was very pleased with herself; her parents were delighted and relieved. Over the course of the hour-long visit she relaxed into play and began to communicate directly with me.

In another example, four-year-old Jacob's parents worried that he might have bipolar disorder. As they tried to tell me about the difficulties at home, he began to escalate out of control, climbing on his father, who was sitting with his mother on the couch, and poking him in the face. Thinking creatively about how to manage the situation, I suggested we take five minutes out of our conversation, inviting his parents to join us on the floor and play. Jacob immediately became calm and focused. When the five minutes were up, I asked him to play on his own, and resumed conversation with his parents. He lasted four minutes—I was timing it on my watch—and again he exploded in agitation and anger, screaming and hitting his mother. This time, drawing on the history they had shared that he loved music, I suggested his mother play a song he liked on her phone. He almost immediately became still and quiet, fully absorbed in listening. I could validate their experience of his rapidly shifting moods and behavior. But having "acted it out" in the office in this kind of free-form play, they could begin to make sense of the shifts. They saw not only how his mood changes related to withdrawal of attention, but also that different approaches could help move him out of these disorganized states. His behavior no longer felt so unpredictable; they no longer felt helpless.

With an expanse of an unstructured hour in which to play, the tension that pervades the initial part of an evaluation often evolves into a feeling of relief and calm. Similar to the play *Dancing Lessons*, our one-hour visit is its own little one-act play. Winnicott writes, "In these highly specialized conditions the individual can come together and exist as a unit, not as a defense against anxiety but as an expression of I am, I am myself, I am alive. From this position everything is creative."

The Physical Space

The healing power of the physical space is evident in the weekly mother-baby group that I described in the last chapter. The large space where the groups are held, with floor-to-ceiling windows, offers opportunity to stretch out and relax. The mothers sit on the floor in a circle with their babies on blankets, in their arms, or asleep in their carriers. Large bouncy balls on the periphery offer opportunity to soothe a crying baby while still participating in the discussion. Often a mom, engrossed in telling a story, will continue without pause as she carries her infant to one of changing tables available in the room. Even the ample parking adds to the sense of space, one less stress in navigating from home to group.

The mothers often come into the room in groups, having begun their sharing conversation in the hallway: "He's been up all night" or "I'm going back to work next week and can hardly stand to think about it" or "My mother-in-law tries to help, but she makes me feel like I don't know what I'm doing."

Over the first fifteen minutes they take time to settle in, unbundling babies in the harshest winter months, holding one another's babies, continuing the easy sharing. The group runs for eight weeks, with an hour and a half for each session, though the time bleeds over the edges before, and after in the rebundling. Mothers continue the conversation over lunch and then online. Babies range in age from weeks to months.

The babies cycle through sleep, alert interaction, fussy periods, crying, and feeding. Their mothers, many of them doing this for the first time, intuitively guide their infants through these multiple transitions while simultaneously engaging in meaningful conversation. The loosely structured format is organized around such topics as navigating relationships with a spouse, going back to work, or sleep challenges. The group leader begins by giving each mother time to talk about the past week. She then gently guides the conversation, offering support and careful listening, when, as inevitably happens, they enter the territory of deep and painful feelings.

"I'm so angry at my husband all the time," one mother began. Yet she was puzzled by her anger, as he was helpful and took the baby as soon as he came home from work, doing what he could to support her. "I can't think of anything different he should be doing, "she said. But she hated these deep feelings of resentment that plagued her. She described constant worrying, revealing a history of severe anxiety for which she was taking medication. "I wonder," I asked, "if you are envious of his lack of anxiety." Tears of recognition began to flow. The group offered quiet and respect, giving her time to process this new understanding. Other mothers shared similar experiences. That mother, by giving words to her feelings about her husband, was able to let go of that debilitating rage, express her true feelings, and begin to make use of the support he was offering.

The mothers, along with the group leader, had set aside these ninety minutes to be fully present with one another and with their babies. When I joined the group as a guest every eight-week cycle, I would find that in that ninety minutes, the rest of the world completely disappeared. The culture of the group reflects a valuing of that space and time for being present—with one another and with their babies.

One group leader articulated this idea well:

As a facilitator of groups for new moms, my goal is to create a safe, welcoming space where mothers can "tell it like it is" and speak candidly about what they're experiencing. Early parenthood brings many highs and lows, and new moms are often bombarded with information and advice about parenting, but have no space to process their feelings and experiences. New moms need that emotional space to talk, vent, process, and express their feelings without judgment from others.

The value of the physical space is recognized by Bright Spaces, a program of the organization Bright Horizons, which builds "warm, safe enriching places" in homeless shelters and other agencies for children in crisis. With cozy nooks and comfortable furniture, Bright Spaces are designed to be engaging, comfortable places for children and families—a place to "build relationships, heal from trauma through play and experience the joy of childhood."

A colleague described her work in one of these spaces with mothers who have experienced domestic violence and are living in homeless shelters with their children. She described "hanging out" with the mothers and children in an effort to "build trust and co-wondering." They covered a range of topics, with many of the moms sharing pregnancy stories. The conversation often turned to "behavior problems" and questions about medication. Many of the mothers were on medication themselves, so it seemed like an inevitable next step for their children.

My colleague described how the physical space itself, designed by Bright Spaces, encourages these moms to feel valued. In this environment of both comfort and understanding, they become curious about the meaning of their children's behavior. She said, "For me what these opportunities of 'hanging out' provide is that safe space for moms to share their story, and begin the think about what their children's story might be."

When Space and Time Are Limited

Our culture of advice and quick fixes may discourage taking the time to hear the full story. This fact was vividly evident in a recent radio interview that was part of a whirlwind PR tour following publication of a children's book on toilet training for which I wrote the parent guide. In the twenty-two interviews over a span of four hours, I explained to my interviewers that it is not a "how to" guide but rather a set of "guiding principles."

In this particular interview, the radio show host, the mom of a three-year-old, spent the bulk of the ten-minute conversation telling me about her frustration with her son's saying no to repeated requests to poop on the potty. As she was not a patient, and the purpose of the conversation was to talk about the book, I repeated the advice from the parent guide, while again qualifying it with the need to recognize that each child-parent pair is unique. I emphasized that the process needs to be tailored not only to each individual child, but also to the family circumstances under which toilet training is occurring.

With about two minutes to go, she mentioned that she was pregnant with twins. After giving me about thirty seconds to address the possible relevance of this fact, she switched to the topic of her husband, who rather than helping by being a model for their son, locks the door to the bathroom to protect his private time. The other radio host, a man, interjected with, "When the twins come, there will be no private time." Now we were getting somewhere. Seconds later came, "Thank you for joining us on our program."

The whole process felt emblematic of the trouble with our culture of advice and quick fixes. If there is an exclusive focus on what to do about "problem behavior," there is no time to reflect on the nuances and complexities of relationships. These relationships, and the family stories they are part of, are inevitably inextricably linked to the "problem." In telling the full story, what to do usually becomes clear.

For the mom of this three-year-old, that might mean backing off from the toilet training until after the babies are born. It might mean that some more explaining about where babies come from is indicated (a three-year-old might very well confuse the babies in the tummy with poop and hold on to the poop in an effort to be like Mom). There might be some work that needs to be done in the marriage in terms of shared responsibility for parenting. An opportunity to listen to the story offers the path to meaningful solutions.

When space and time are limited, I find myself needing to think creatively. Both were in short supply in my job at a local community health center, where many families struggle with generations of poverty, mental illness, and sometimes neglect and abuse. In that setting as the behavioral pediatrician, I had a tiny office that was not only often unbearably hot, especially with children and parents crammed in, sitting on the floor to play, but the walls were so thin that we could hear the conversations of the office staff on the other side. Here were the families with the greatest need, in a space that gave little consideration to comfort and safety.

Twelve-year-old Sara was scheduled for a fifty-minute "ADHD evaluation." Both the health center and the family expected I would provide an answer to the question "Does she have ADHD?" and also a plan for treatment. Sara came into my office with her mother, Maxine, who immediately began to berate her in an angry tone. "She never listens. She's defiant. She's terrible—all over the place. I know she has that ADHD thing and needs medication." Sara sunk into her seat and withdrew into the hood of her jacket in the face of her mother's attack. In that small space she made her best effort to disappear.

I took a deep breath, thinking on my feet of a way to rescue the situation within the fifty minutes. The room felt literally too small to contain the powerful feelings, mostly of rage directed at Sara. My first step was to ask her mother to wait in the waiting room, literally to give Sara some space. I did not expect her to tell me what was wrong, but without her mother there she responded to my interest by sitting up and answering my general questions about school. Once I saw that she had begun to relax, I had her mother come back in the room.

Limited by the small space, I positioned myself in a way that indicated I was ready to hear Maxine's whole story, and expressed curiosity about when the difficulties started. I sat angled between mother and daughter so that I could convey interest in both. I made a conscious effort to slow things down and to simply be present in the moment.

Maxine too seemed to relax and her angry demeanor softened. She responded by opening up. She first told of a traumatic fire a few years earlier that had forced the family (she had two younger children) to be homeless for a number of months. She had been terrified that she would be accused of neglect and that her children would be taken away, so she hadn't, until now, spoken about the episode. Then, perhaps responding to my nonjudgmental attitude, she went on. She told me of another traumatic fire when she was a child. Then she spoke of her own struggles with serious mental illness and her trouble finding help for herself.

While Maxine spoke, Sara relaxed and the hood came off. About twenty minutes into the story, Maxine turned to her daughter and said tearfully, "It's probably been hard for you to see me like this." And then to me, "I think she misses me." Maxine now saw her daughter's behavior not as "difficult" but as a way to connect with her.

By making the choice within our limited time not to ask questions about symptoms of ADHD, but rather to listen to the story, I was able to offer an opportunity for a meaningful moment of connection between parent and child. But, for reasons I will explore in detail in the following chapter, our current health-care system does not support this kind of listening. The pressures, given the lack of this space and time, to diagnose and medicate, may be too great.

Beyond Reassurance

A great teacher of mine, child psychiatrist Michael Jellinek, once said to me, "Reassurance is an assault." When a parent is worried that something is wrong, worried enough to seek help, often repeatedly, reassurance that "everything is fine" can be experienced as a kind of disconnect, a way of being dismissed or misunderstood. In this situation, space and time to discover meaning can be critical.

Maria, mother of four-month-old Elena, called to make an appointment in my behavioral pediatrics practice. Her thick accent—I placed it as Eastern European—made it difficult for me to understand her concern over the phone. She arrived at my office with her husband, Alexander, who spoke little English. Although I had a blanket on the floor covered with toys, Maria stood tentatively, her movements awkward and hesitant, until I suggested she put Elena down.

Immediately Elena gave me a huge grin, kicking her little legs that her mother had, with my gentle encouragement, released from her snowsuit. At first Maria sat tensely on a chair, not joining us on the floor, speaking in a somewhat remote and intellectual tone, while she told me her story. I played with Elena, smiling with her as I observed that she liked to be held in a standing position to better see the world. Maria eventually joined us on the floor, but did not join me in playing with Elena.

Maria was fully absorbed in describing a scary moment just after Elena's birth, when she had needed some oxygen. Elena had been in the special care nursery for about an hour before she was reunited with her mother. Multiple doctors had reassured Maria that Elena was fine. She had seen her regular pediatrician for checkups, and he had expressed no concerns about Elena's development. Yet Maria was convinced that there was something wrong with her brain. Specifically with her ability to relate to other people—it was her social development that Maria was worried about.

Puzzled by the incongruity between this delightful healthy baby and this anxious, unengaged mom, I watched the story unfold so that I might make sense of it. About halfway through the visit, Elena began to fuss. Alexander swooped in from his position on the periphery of the room and immediately began to give Elena a bottle. She continued to fuss, her father making repeated efforts to force the bottle in her mouth while Maria helplessly looked on. Now I began to put the pieces together. Maria had told me that she was the breadwinner, and worked long hours. Alexander had been a practicing physician in their home country, but he had not gotten his US medical license, and so was Elena's primary caregiver.

As Elena continued to fuss, I asked Maria whether she perhaps knew what would soothe the baby. When Alexander moved in, she had withdrawn again, getting up from the floor and sitting stiffly in a chair. When I encouraged her to take the baby, she stood and made motions toward Alexander and Elena. I stood with them. The three of us were now standing in our socks. Even when Elena was in her mother's arms, Alexander continued to make efforts to grab the baby back. I shared my observation that Alexander, likely because he was used to having primary responsibility, seemed inclined to take over without giving Maria space to figure things out with her daughter. But she had a different interpretation of his behavior. "He thinks I don't know how to take care of her."

I now had a better understanding of the situation. Elena had been a fussy baby until she was about eight weeks old, just the time when Maria had gone back to work. They had never gotten a chance to learn to read each other's signals. "I wonder if you miss Elena," I said. Immediately her eyes filled with tears. Her whole posture changed. Words poured out as she shared her feelings of terrible inadequacy. She described her heartache and humiliation going to a mother-baby group where the other mothers seemed to know exactly how to respond to their infants, and she felt unsure and helpless. As she spoke, she stood with Elena in her arms, walking around the space and gently rocking her. Elena quieted and again smiled, this time at her mother.

Maria was not worried about Elena's social development, but rather Elena's connection specifically with her. It took this setting and this hour when we were free to move around and "play" to come to this new understanding.

Maria came to the visit with a stance of defensiveness that was most likely completely out of her awareness. I did not ask her questions but instead let the experience of being with me, with an expanse of time to relax, allow her to let her defenses down. But it did not take much time. By forty minutes into the visit there was a profound transformation in the bodies of both mother and daughter as they relaxed into each other. While Alexander was limited by language, he, too, seemed relieved that his wife was happy.

While we were not measuring heart rate or blood pressure, we could see the change in physiology reflected in Maria's change in posture, in the way she held her body. That stiff, awkward stance gave way to natural movement. We both stood, Maria facing me and looking directly at me as she gently rocked her baby.

Within the first five minutes of the visit I could tell that Elena was a normal, healthy baby. But Maria was not ready to hear it. What seemed to me an "irrational" worry was actually her brain's defensive response in the face of overwhelming shame. She was unable to engage the higher cortical centers of her brain responsible for rational thought. It is possible that, under control of the "primitive vagus" that takes over when a person feels threatened, Maria could not hear the doctors' reassurances. I needed to offer her space and time to let those defenses down.

Alexander remained on the periphery of this dance. He made a few attempts to take Elena from her mother and I gently encouraged him to give her some time. My understanding of the situation was that Maria had not had a chance to learn her own dance with Elena. She needed to experience the normal "disruption and repair," as described by Ed Tronick, to develop her own relationship with her daughter. When her husband, with the best of intentions, swooped in to take the baby whenever she fussed, Maria and Elena lost the opportunity.

I observed with Maria that what she was experiencing is a common phenomenon for fathers. When mothers are the primary caregivers, they may claim to "know the baby best" and so not give fathers a chance. Here the situation was reversed, and made even more painful because of the expectation that as the mother she should instinctively know how to comfort her baby.

I suggested that she share our observations with Alexander at home, when they could speak their native language. She would ask him to give her a chance to comfort Elena before grabbing her away.

I learned, when I saw them a few weeks later, that Maria had changed a lot more in her life than the way she cared for her baby. That one-hour visit had provided the energy to transform this young family. Maria had changed her schedule, working fewer hours so that she could spend more time with Elena. Alexander had gotten a job, not as a physician, but he was willing to take a lesser job to help support the family if it would benefit the relationship between his wife and daughter. During our visit, Maria had an opportunity to feel her connection with her daughter, and feel the pain of that lost connection. She saw that she did not want to live her life like that. During our follow-up visit Maria's confidence had increased dramatically. Her worries that there was "something wrong" with her daughter had vanished.

In a shorter appointment, with a focus on just the baby and whether she had a problem, it is unlikely that the family and I would have found ourselves to this place of understanding that brought with it connection, healing, and growth.

Listening and Being Heard

Some of my pediatrician colleagues respond to this emphasis on the significance of time in healing with outrage. Not that they disagree, but in their day-to-day practice time for listening may be nonexistent. Primary care practices must have a large staff to manage the complexities of multiple different insurance plans. Office managers spend hours making calls and filling out forms to get insurance companies to give what is known as "prior authorization" for such things as MRIs, neuropsychological testing, and referrals to specialists. A recent study showed that prior authorization consumes twenty hours a week for an average medical practice. For the practice to be viable and support this staff, the doctors are forced to see more patients in less time.

Giving space and time to parents, where they can speak in a safe environment, sometimes without the child present, is essential for listening to children. In our current health-care system, the reimbursement structure may be an obstacle to listening to parents, as visits are billed under the child's name. After doing some research, I learned that if I wrote in my note that the child was not present due to the nature of the material discussed, I would be reimbursed for visits with parents alone. However, many clinicians are unaware of, or do not make use of, this opportunity. While I always aim to see both parents alone without the child in a full-hour initial evaluation, this practice is the exception. It is not uncommon for diagnoses to be made and medication prescribed with input only from one parent, usually the mother. During one of the weekends of Dr. Tronick's Infant Parent Mental Health training program, one young social worker spoke to the group about agonizing visits where a mother described her feelings of rage at her child's father, and her own history of trauma, while her three-year-old son played at her feet, clearly taking in every word. This clinician felt helplessly trapped by the reimbursement structure into providing care in a way that she recognized was wrong.

At a point in my career when I was forging new territory and so had few colleagues with whom to discuss the sometimes-difficult work, I called a friend who is an experienced psychoanalyst. I explained this feeling of professional isolation and asked whether we could talk. "Perhaps we could meet for coffee?" I said. Although we were friends, and might have done this in a more casual way, he insisted that I make an appointment and set aside a full fifty minutes. When we were settled in, he pointed out how I had not given myself the time needed, but rather was shortchanging myself by suggesting we squeeze in these important conversations. "You can't be there for others," he wisely told me, "unless you take care of yourself." When as a general pediatrician, I was aware of a waiting room of patients who would all be upset and angry if I spent more than the allotted fifteen minutes with the distraught mother in front of me, my mind was not available for listening.

Looking Ahead to Solutions

A pediatrician colleague, Howard King, runs a wonderful program, the Children's Emotional HealthLink (CEHL), whose cornerstone is listening to pediatricians to fortify their efforts to listen to parents. This listening in turn serves to support parent-child relationships and promote mental health. Participants in the program meet monthly over a year in an intimate setting where they develop trusting relationships and opportunity to share their struggles as professionals, including the way their patients' stories resonate with their own personal stories. CEHL, as described on the website, "is dedicated to helping parents, pediatricians, and other providers improve the emotional health of children and families. CEHL provides information designed to empower parents and to assist pediatricians to reach out to children and families in need."

Primary care clinicians have regular contact with young children and families often over years. But they may have neither adequate training nor adequate time to deal with the problems they are ideally situated to identify and treat. Issues in families and relationships that, if addressed early, may prevent later mental health problems, may go unrecognized. Psychiatric training emphasizing treatment of established psychiatric disorders. In the current system, in which the pediatrician may not have the time or training, and the child psychiatrist is trained in a disease model that emphasizes diagnosing disorders and prescribing of medication, prevention falls through the cracks.

I recently had the opportunity to teach a seminar on infant mental health to the child psychiatry fellows at a major teaching hospital. After spending an hour giving an overview of contemporary research in infant mental health, I presented a case of a seven-year-old boy with a very complex family and developmental history. I then turned to the group and asked how they would make sense of his behavior. A fellow responded without pause, "I would see if he met *DSM* diagnostic criteria for a mood disorder and then consider prescribing an SSRI." A similarly complex case was met by this question from the head of child psychiatry: "Do the parents need parent training or does the child have ADHD and need medication?"

Psychiatrists trained in the age of biological psychiatry have grown up in a professional family with a language of "disorder" that has likely shaped the way they think. Making the shift to listen to a story in a way that leads to discovery of the meaning of behavior in developmental context, especially when they too are pressed for time, may be difficult. Education about new research and knowledge of the science of child development needs to be incorporated from the start into training for professionals who work with children and families.

The growing number of professionals trained in early childhood mental health can fill this crack in the system where missed opportunities now fall. A specialist trained in this way situated directly in the primary care setting, where families come for well child care, can make room for prevention. The Healthy Steps[SM] program, developed by Margot Kaplan-Sanoff and colleagues, is one example. This model normalizes the struggles of parents and children, and reduces the risk of being labeled with a mental health disorder. My colleagues and I often refer to a "nice lady [or man] down the hall model." Such a person can take the time to listen to the story and set the family on a better path. This kind of integration of mental health care into primary care, in contrast to a psychiatry model that simply supports doctors in diagnosing disorders and prescribing medication, is a true model of prevention.

Throughout these stories runs an image of holding, containing, as in Russian dolls. When helping professionals feel supported in using their time to listen, they are more likely to be fully present to hear a parent's story. Feeling recognized and understood, parents are then freed to be fully present with a child, to offer that holding environment that is central to healthy growth and development.

In contrast, as we will see in the following section, a pervasive experience of feeling unheard is common. When children, parents, friends, spouses, and professionals are not listening, it is most often because they themselves feel overwhelmed. If we fail to act to protect space and time for listening, the consequences for the next generation may be devastating.

Part Three

The Silencing
of Children

Six

The Rush to Label and Medicate

In the introductory chapter of his book *The Doctor, His Patient and the Illness*, psychoanalyst Michael Balint writes that "it was not only the bottle of medicine or box of pills that mattered, but the way the doctor gave them to the patient—in fact, the whole atmosphere in which the drug was given and taken."

An article about the placebo effect, based on the work of Harvard professor Ted J. Kaptchuk, makes a similar point: "Wise doctors and nurses . . . have found, usually just by personal experience, that their 'everything else'—respect, attention, comfort, empathy, touch—often does the lion's share of medical care, no deception required. Sometimes the prescription is just the afterthought." One can understand the placebo effect as a form of listening. By prescribing a pill, the doctor communicates: "I hear you and recognize your suffering."

Under the influence of the pharmaceutical and health insurance industries this issue has gotten turned on its head. The pill itself is seen as the primary treatment, and the relationship—the respectful, careful listening—is relegated to "everything else."

Recently I received in the mail, in exchange for filling out a questionnaire about a study of diversion—the use of ADHD medications by individuals for whom it was not prescribed—a pretty laminated poster of all the drugs currently available for treatment of ADHD.

Looking at the poster, I wondered about the paradox of the parallel increase in availability of new psychiatric drugs—I counted twenty-two different formulations for ADHD medications on that poster—and the rise of serious mental health problems. Could it be that the drugs themselves are responsible for this increase? Serious mental health problems in the college community are growing at rapid rates. If the drugs were effective in childhood, shouldn't we see a significant *decline* in serious mental illness in college?

I'm not speaking about the unknown long-term effects of these medications themselves on the growing brain, though certainly that is an important question. A survey of close to two thousand people being prescribed antidepressants showed a much higher than expected rate of serious psychological side effects. Almost half described "feeling emotionally numb" and "caring less about others." Rather, I am wondering whether the way psychiatric diagnoses and medication have replaced listening is linked to the rise in mental illness. Many factors in our health-care system drive the increase in prescriptions, which may be inextricably linked with lost opportunity not only for prevention of mental illness, but also for fostering of strength and resilience.

A recent report showed that close to 1 in 3 students who first seek help from college counseling services is already on medication. At a conference exploring this escalating use of psychiatric medication, nine participating college counseling centers observed that many students have an expectation that "disturbing feelings were to be 'managed' generally via medication, rather than learned from." Conference leader M. Gerard Fromm, in his description of the conference findings, writes, "Students also arrive with less perspective on development, less experience with how to talk about themselves, and less recognition of the importance of relationships in their lives."

Prescribing of psychiatric medication is a common endpoint of multiple social forces. Pressures on primary care clinicians, shortage of qualified mental health professionals, and aggressive marketing by the pharmaceutical industry are some of the factors that have converged to support a culture in which medication is routinely prescribed without time spent with patients to listen and understand their problems.

The influence of the health insurance industry is equally significant. It is more profitable to cover a brief "medication check" than a fifty-minute visit. Prescribing medication takes much less time than sitting with people until they trust you enough to talk about what is important in their lives. In a dramatic example of the tail wagging the dog, the need to get services "covered" by insurance may drive families and physicians to seek a diagnosis of a disorder, leading a child on a path to medication. Patricia Wen, a *Boston Globe* reporter who brilliantly exposed the way the system of supplemental security income (SSI) for disabilities incentivizes diagnosis of mental illness in children, reported in 2014 that for families living in poverty, disability income, mainly for behavioral, emotional, and learning disorders, surpassed welfare as the primary source of financial support.

In my conversations with pediatricians on the front lines, I find most are stymied by these pressures. When we are overwhelmed in the face of time constraints, many of us go into survival mode, with the immediate aim just to get through the day. Primary care clinicians may find themselves prescribing medication because they feel they have no other options.

One colleague bemoaned the fact that in light of her inability to address the family dynamics and socio-economic circumstances "all she has available" is medications to help with the child's symptoms. She described patients who come from unstable environments, where parents are themselves stressed and overwhelmed. She recognized that children's "difficult," "impulsive," "oppositional" behavior is a communication about stressors that are making families less competent at caring for them. However, she lacked the resources or the time to lessen these overwhelming stressors. Feeling helpless, she used the only resource she had, medication. When she could bear to think about it, she recognized that medication was just shutting off children's efforts to tell her something—in effect silencing their voices.

Mental health professionals are similarly squeezed by the system. Many do not take insurance because the number of hoops these companies require them and their patients to jump through, in parallel with ever-decreasing payments, has skyrocketed. Those who continue to participate in insurance plans tell horror stories of battles to get approval for ongoing therapy with patients. For example, one social worker told me that when patients in our community receiving Medicaid were suddenly switched from one insurance plan to another, she and her colleagues had to scramble to get on to this new plan, with reams of paperwork and success in no way guaranteed, to be able to continue work with patients they had been treating for years.

Psychiatric nurse practitioners, whose primary job is often to prescribe medication, also express frustrations with a system that places so little value on listening. In mental health care centers, therapists who do not prescribe medication may feel undermined when they are told to check with the prescribers if there is an escalation in a patient's symptoms. Those who do prescribe receive frequent requests from schools to adjust a child's medication because she is "acting up." Often a "med eval" is the first step, and only after that is there a secondary step, a referral for therapy if the prescriber thinks it is called for. One psychiatric nurse practitioner spoke of feeling great pressure to continually eliminate problem behavior with medication. She worried about the message this is sending to families.

Multiple drugs (polypharmacy) are increasingly used for treatment of mental health problems in children, not only by psychiatrists but also by primary care clinicians who are not specifically trained in treatment of psychiatric illness. Use of atypical antipsychotics, such as risperidone, in very young children, has doubled, despite the fact that these drugs are not approved by the FDA for patients younger than age five. The chief of child psychiatry at a well-respected Boston teaching hospital recently told me, when I was concerned about its use in a four-year-old girl, that "antipsychotics are as safe as asthma drugs." While asthma medications (which have their own side effects) have been around for decades, we have sparse data on use of these powerful antipsychotic medications, especially in young children. They are known to cause not only significant weight gain, but also changes in the endocrine system, with rising rates of diabetes and other metabolic syndromes. Nevertheless, aggressive marketing of these medications and prescribing for a wide range of uses continues to rise.

Medicating Children to Sleep

Treatment of sleep problems in childhood is a vivid example of the way our current system of care misses opportunities for prevention by treating the symptom, rather than taking time to understand what the behavior is communicating. Despite the fact that no sleep medications are approved for use in children, a study published in the journal *Sleep Medicine* revealed that most child psychiatrists prescribe such drugs for sleep at least once a month. The study was funded by Sanofi-Aventis, makers of Ambien. One might say sleep medications are a Band-Aid, but unfortunately they are not nearly as benign. Apart from their side effects, they may hide a disrupted relationship.

Sleep problems in children involve both parent and child. However, using medication places the "problem" squarely in the child. By condoning this treatment, we may not hear what is behind the conflict, and miss an opportunity to support and mend parent-child relationships.

For children, sleep patterns follow a typical developmental progression, and sleep issues can only be understood in developmental context. In infancy a child learns what are commonly called sleep associations. The breast, a pacifier, a lovey, or even a parent's hair may be what a child associates with falling asleep. Frequent night waking, expected by parents in the early weeks and months, can become a problem if that sleep association involves a parent's physical presence. As the months wear on, parents become severely sleep deprived, and often find that this pattern is not so easy to change.

In toddlerhood, as a child in a normal healthy way begins to assert her independence, she may resist bedtime. Rather than focusing on "making a child go to bed," addressing this aspect of sleep disruption involves looking at the way parent and child may be locked in battles for control that extend well beyond bedtime. The act of going to sleep, even if the child is in the same room or bed, represents a separation. A child who handles the first day of preschool with grace may suddenly refuse to go to bed, or begin waking during the night.

Managing sleep is one of the great challenges of being a parent. It can be fraught with complex ambivalent feelings. When parents come to see me for "problem behavior" in a child, hearing about family sleep habits is an essential step in making sense of the problem. When children have difficulty with regulating their emotions, calm necessary to fall asleep may be not come easily. Sleep deprivation, in turn, makes emotional regulation more challenging, leading to a vicious cycle, where both parent and child can become increasingly irritable and agitated.

Many children I see with a diagnosis of ADHD have been engaging in battles with their parents for years around sleep, compounded by a range of conflicts within the family. Sleep disruption often is a cause, rather than result, of attention problems. Consider fifteen-year-old Sarah, who came to me with a diagnosis of ADHD, made by her previous physician. I learned that until she was thirteen, her mother lay in bed with her every night until she fell asleep. Then on the day of her birthday, her mother decided that her daughter was too old for this habit and abruptly stopped, insisting that she fall asleep on her own. Not surprisingly, Sarah's brain and body had no idea how to fall asleep independently, so she was staying up until two or three o'clock every morning, sneaking her laptop into bed with her. Her inattentiveness during the day was due in large part to her chronic severe sleep deprivation, which in turn resulted from troubles in her relationship with her mother.

A recent study that received a lot of media attention, with such news articles as "More Sleep Might Help Tots Tantrums," showed that children who slept fewer than 9.4 hours had more impulsivity, anger, tantrums, and annoying behavior. While this study is important because it calls attention to the need to address sleep in the setting of behavior problems, simple admonitions to have a child get more sleep are not only unhelpful, but may also make parents feel worse.

I feel for the parent who reads an article recommending that a child get more sleep to improve behavior, and is unable to change the situation because the underlying cause is not addressed. This is where our culture of advice and quick fixes can lead parents to be overwhelmed by feelings of inadequacy and guilt. The original article describes an "association" between lack of sleep and behavior problems. But it is not a simple cause and effect. Sleep problems are behavior problems. To know the cause, or what the behavior is communicating, one must know the family story.

There are many ways healthy sleep patterns can get derailed. For example, ideally parents make a conscious choice about whether they want their baby to sleep separately in a different room. But often parents don't agree, or they just take the path of least resistance. In these circumstances a child in the bed can cause significant stress and marital discord. Another common scenario is when a parent—a father or a mother—struggles with depression. Sleep deprivation will aggravate symptoms, which often include irritability. When a parent is quick to lash out, a child may become anxious. Sometimes this anxiety leads to acting out, in the form of oppositional behavior. A two-year-old doesn't know how to say, "I need you to be with me and I feel sad when you are angry." While it may seem illogical, she may simply see that when she is "difficult," her parents are more engaged with her. Bedtime refusal and frequent night waking are common expressions of separation anxiety.

If a family together with a pediatrician or therapist take the time, then it is possible to make sense of the situation, to strengthen relationships and set the whole family on a better path. The younger the child, the easier this is to do.

I first saw Charles when he was two years old. His mother, Donna, described terribly disrupted sleep. He would wake multiple times at night and scream for her. Even as she held him and tried to reassure him with her presence, he would continue to thrash and cry out. His behavior was so wild and out of control that his parents feared he was having a seizure. Donna was mystified when he screamed for her even though she was right next to him. To reassure both them and myself, I sent him to a neurologist who, after an exam and EEG, declared that there was nothing wrong. He prescribed a tricyclic antidepressant.

His mother threw the pamphlet about the drug in the garbage and arrived at my office horrified, yet ready to do the work of addressing their problem in a meaningful way.

Charles had been a "difficult" baby since birth. He cried easily and needed a lot of help to settle. He certainly had his part to play in the development of this problem. But when Donna had time to tell her story, we were able to understand her role in these disrupted nights. When she was a young child, her own mother, who had severe mental illness, had abandoned Donna. Not only had she been left alone in her crib for long periods as an infant, but also as Donna grew up, her mother had not been emotionally available to her, though she had provided physical care. Donna recognized that in order to be emotionally available to Charles in the way he needed, she would have to address her own trauma.

Donna came to understand that Charles's neediness at bedtime was so disturbing to her that emotionally she was not there, though physically she was present. She experienced his needy behavior as threatening because it provoked fearful memories of her own traumatic loss. But her maternal instinct would not let the fight-or-flight response take over; she would neither hit nor abandon Charles. Her emotional absence, however, was unconsciously betrayed by her face and voice, likely under the influence of the primitive vagus, as I described in Chapter 5. As we know, children may be highly attuned to our emotional state. Charles's sensitivity was heightened by the ongoing daytime battles, both cause and result of severe sleep deprivation.

Once this pattern was brought in to awareness through the telling of her story, Donna's unconscious response became conscious and so she was able to change it. Feeling supported and understood, she was better able to be emotionally present with Charles at bedtime and through the episodes of night waking. Donna recognized the way her own experience was affecting her parenting and that she might need to revisit this early loss. But the pressing issue of sleep deprivation could be addressed more immediately.

When parents come to see me after weeks, months, or even years of turmoil around sleep, both parent and child have a heightened state of arousal simply thinking about the coming night. It can take some time for the body to re-equilibrate so that both parent and child can feel calm with the approach of bedtime. But once the meaning of the behavior is understood, a positive cycle can be set in place. When parents don't dread bedtime, daytime relationships also usually improve. For Charles and Donna, with mother and child reconnecting, gradually the sleep disruption subsided.

An innovative pediatric practice in Portland, Oregon, uses the ACE score that I described in Chapter 4 to uncover the issues in a parent's history that may impact a child's development. In a blog post about the program, Jane Ellen Stevens, who writes extensively about application of the ACE study, describes a story similar to that of Charles and Donna. After implementing the ACE score into the practice, one pediatrician learns from her patient's mother that her own mother abandoned her at the age of two. This mother tells her doctor that her baby's crying "triggered a lot of fear." Her first child had a lot of sleep problems, and when this story came out in a visit for her second infant, her pediatrician understood why the advice she had given this mother hadn't worked. Once this story had been told, however, they could have a more meaningful and useful discussion about managing sleep with this new baby.

I once listened to a conversation among a group of child psychiatrists about treatment of "insomnia" in a five-year-old. Back and forth they went about various drugs—melatonin, Benadryl, clonidine, Trazodone—with discussion focused on dose and medication interactions. When one psychiatrist recommended risperidone, not approved for use in children for any reason and certainly not for sleep disruption, I joined the conversation.

"Has a developmental sleep history already been done?" I asked hopefully. "Has the child ever learned to fall asleep independently?" I explained that I find it useful to break sleep problems down into three components—sleep associations, independence and control issues, and separation issues, and then address the problem in reverse order, treating the separation anxiety, the need for limit setting, and last the sleep associations. Clearly this child had experienced a lot of significant disruptions (her mother was seriously mentally ill), but I still wondered whether an in-depth understanding of the sleep problem could lead to effective treatment without medication.

While some others in the conversation suggested behavior management techniques for "sleep hygiene," the psychiatrist advocating for risperidone then pointed to a quality-of-life issue. He said it would be better for the whole family if the child could sleep. I agreed.

I told them that I was not thinking of "sleep hygiene" or behavior management as much as getting an understanding of the developmental origins of the sleep problem. "Insomnia" is not an adequate explanation. I'm not even sure what it means for a young child. Even in a family where a parent has serious mental illness, efforts to make sense of a child's behavior can lead to meaningful solutions. In the setting of long-term bedtime refusal and sleep disruption, often there has been a lot of yelling during the night, and everyone is highly agitated around bedtime every day. If the child has never learned to fall asleep independently, some form of co-sleeping may have a role to play until the situation is calmed down. Or, if a mother herself is severely sleep deprived, as is often the case, perhaps she needs some kind of respite care for a few days to get uninterrupted sleep. Once both parent and child have slept for several nights, the problem will have a different feel and less sense of urgency, allowing parents and caregivers to explore solutions. In the face of sleep problems, the lack of time for listening and understanding, together with the use of drugs, is a dangerous combination.

Foster Care, Shoes, and Antipsychotics

An alarming recent study showed that antipsychotics, such as risperidone, are being prescribed to nearly one third of children in foster care who are diagnosed with ADHD. While there is a range of reasons for a child to be in foster care, one can assume that there has, at minimum, been some experience of trauma and loss. This might include physical and/or emotional abuse. Given what we know about intergenerational transmission of abuse and neglect, it is also quite likely that the abusing or neglectful biological parent was herself subject to some form of developmental trauma.

This statistic about foster children brought to mind a common complaint I hear from parents about putting on shoes to go out of the house. This kind of scene likely plays out in some form in every household with a young child. A child will dawdle, ignoring multiple requests. The situation will escalate to the point where the parent becomes increasingly angry and frustrated, and the child descends into an all-out tantrum. This typical and very ordinary interaction can be useful to keep in mind as we aim to understand why a child who is in foster care might exhibit behavior that calls for bringing out pharmaceutical big guns.

Young children inevitably have tantrums, a normal healthy part of development. But when a child's behavior, as they say, pushes our buttons, parents may be unable to think clearly. They may become overwhelmed with rage, or shut down emotionally. In efforts to protect the child from anger, a dissociative response may take over. For the child, it is as if her parent suddenly isn't there. But usually the moment passes, the child calms down, and the parent returns. The disruption is repaired.

With a neglectful and/or abusive parent, when a child has a developmentally normal tantrum, her parent may dissociate and not return. Psychologist Ed Tronick references "The Good, the Bad and the Ugly" to capture the range of parent-child interactions. The "good" are the typical rifts and repairs in daily interactions; the "bad," a greater than average frequency of these, such as occur when parent and child are engaged in a longer-term struggle. The "ugly" occurs in situations of abuse and neglect, when there is no opportunity to repair the mismatch. In this situation, a child learns that her own emotional distress may lead to abandonment. If this pattern of interaction occurs over a period of time, she may, in an adaptive response, meet her parent's dissociation with her own form of dissociation.

Now put this same child in foster care, with a nonabusing caregiver, and ask her to put on her shoes to go outside. She may be involved in play and have some perfectly reasonable explanation for refusing. But what starts out as a typical parent-child interaction, in which a parent expresses her own frustration and disappointment, can quickly lead a foster child into wildly out-of-control behavior. The child's own distress makes her anticipate another abandonment by a caregiver. So, in a protective way, she may dissociate. I've heard parents whose adopted children have experienced early trauma say, "It's like she's not even there." Out of context, this behavior may look, as I have heard from many bewildered foster and adoptive parents, "crazy."

But how do these children get the ADHD diagnosis? Psychoanalyst Robert Furman offers an alternate way to understand behavior that is called ADHD. He describes how when children experience intolerable emotional distress, they have a range of options. They may withdraw into fantasy—distractibility and inattention; use actions, rather than words—hyperactivity; or express outbursts of rage—irritability. When not listening extends to other arenas besides the home, teachers, parents, and clinicians may reframe this behavior as "not paying attention." Impulsivity also often accompanies both neglect and abuse. When children have not been held in mind, they do not develop the ability to think about feelings, and impulsive behavior is one result. These behaviors may, according to checklists commonly used to make the diagnosis, then be labeled as ADHD when in fact they represent not a disorder, but an adaptive response to an overwhelming experience. Putting these two scenarios together, we can understand how children in foster care end up labeled with ADHD and eventually put on antipsychotic medication.

This approach essentially puts a muzzle on the child. The child's behavior is a form of communication. It says, "I have never learned how to manage myself in the face of life's inevitable frustrations." Rather than silence her with a powerful drug that is well known to have serious side effects, we need to listen to that communication.

Even in less extreme circumstances, without abuse and neglect or placement in foster care, we may see similar outcomes. In the setting of mismatches, miscommunications, and misunderstandings, children may develop similar patterns of behavior. In a young child, when we take the time, we can easily recognize this process and set things on a better path. As we have seen, often parents feel terrible shame about both their own and their child's behavior and tell the full story only when they feel safe in a therapeutic relationship.

In my practice I find that for young children monthly visits over a period of three to six months can result in meaningful shifts in relationships accompanied by significant improvement in behavior. I alternate hour-long visits with the parents alone where they can tell their story in a safe environment, with visits with parents and child together where specific behaviors can be discussed in real time as we experience them in the room. Underlying issues, such as marital conflict, parental mental illness or substance abuse, sensory processing issues in the child (see Chapter 8), and unmourned loss (see Chapter 9), can then emerge and be addressed, with referrals made for other forms of treatment when necessary.

Once a child is older, and may have received psychiatric diagnoses and been treated with medication, the story becomes harder to understand. More time and effort is needed to get to the developmental roots of the problem. When this does not happen, medications are adjusted and altered and the original problem is increasingly difficult to identify.

The first step is to recognize the meaning of the behavior. Parents and clinicians are then in a better position to think creatively, as I explore in detail in Chapter 8, about helping a child learn to regulate herself in the face of frustration. At first this might be in a very physical way. For example, she might need to be held in a firm and loving embrace. Or she might need to run around the room. Or hit a punching bag. She might need a soft and gentle voice, rather than a harsh and angry one. As a child gets older, regulating activities, such as dance, theater, and martial arts, can have a significant role to play. Once a child has developed the ability to regulate her body in the face of distress, she can begin, perhaps in the setting of psychotherapy, to give words to her experience. But if we simply silence her with medication, this lost opportunity may restrict her future.

Where Is the Elephant?

In the play and film *God of Carnage*, a witty farce about family life, two couples meet in an elegant living room for an ostensibly civilized conversation about the aggressive act of one couple's child against the other's. The meeting soon degenerates to reveal the underbelly of conflict in the two marriages. Husbands and wives hurl insults, precious items, and even themselves with escalating rage. We see, as they attempt in vain to focus on the children's behavior, the proverbial "elephant in the room."

When I saw the play, it brought to mind another elephant image, presented by the pharmaceutical industry. An issue of the *Journal of Developmental and Behavioral Pediatrics* featured a two-page advertisement from Shire, a company that sells drugs commonly used for treatment of ADHD. A mother and her son sit at the desk of a doctor in a white coat. Behind them is a large elephant draped in a red blanket on which is printed the words *resentful, defiant, angry*. The ad recommends that these symptoms, in addition to the more common symptoms of inattention and hyperactivity, should be addressed. The message is clear: doctors should be treating these symptoms with medication.

After over twenty-five years of practicing pediatrics, during which I sit on the floor, not in a white coat, and play with children, I believe that the depiction of the nature of the elephant in *God of Carnage* is much more accurate and meaningful than that of the pharmaceutical industry. In the play, the elephant is the environment of rage and conflict in which the aggression occurs, while in the ad the elephant is the child's behavior or "symptom."

A recent study, one that supports the drug company's portrayal of the elephant, compared two treatments of aggression in the context of psychiatric diagnosis: "basic therapy" consisting of stimulant medication and parent training, and what they call "augmented therapy," these two treatments plus the antipsychotic risperidone. Neither option asked the questions "What is the child angry about?" "What is behind the child's aggression?" Many of the study's authors have multiple ties to the pharmaceutical industry.

Consider these two stories from my behavioral pediatrics practice. On the phone when she made the appointment, Alicia told me that with six-year-old Mark, everything was a battle. She said, "I need to know what to do to make him listen." As is usual in my practice, I asked her to come for the first visit with Mark's father, Richard, but without Mark. I set up appointments in this way so parents are comfortable to say things they would not want their child to hear. But despite my clear instructions, Alicia came with Mark and without Richard. I was hesitant to proceed, and considered rescheduling, but she seemed desperate, so we decided to go ahead.

While Mark sat on the floor and played, his mother unleashed a string of furious complaints about his terrible behavior. Uneasy about this situation, I tried to deflect this negative attention by asking about Richard and why he was not at the visit. While at first she told me the superficial reason, as she visibly relaxed, she shared a story of constant vicious fighting between herself and her husband. As she spoke, Mark, who had been playing calmly and quietly, took a marker and slowly and deliberately made a black smudge on the yellow wall. His mother was too distracted by her own distress to stop him. I felt that I needed to help them both. I said gently, "You cannot draw on the wall, but maybe you are upset about what we are talking about." He came and sat on his mother's lap. She reluctantly revealed her suspicion that his angry behavior was a reflection of the rage he experienced at home. She saw in that moment not only how the fighting was affecting her son, but also how their concerns about Mark were serving to distract them from their troubled marriage.

Jane's parents, Barbara and Martin, came to see me when her aggressive behavior began to spill over into school. Her third grade teacher told them that not only was she distracted and fidgety, but she seemed increasingly angry. She was referred to me for ADHD evaluation and possible medication. Our first two visits, with just Jane's parents and then together with Jane, were uneventful, as they remained focused on specifics of Jane's behavior. But then Martin called and requested a third visit for him and his wife alone. He had been plagued by feelings of guilt that he wanted to share. He became tearful as he described his cruel and abusive father. He acknowledged being overwhelmed with anger at Jane when she didn't listen. He yelled at her and threatened her. He feared that her behavior was in large part due to the stress of his uncontrolled rage. He longed for a positive role model to learn how to discipline her in a different way. He recognized that he needed help to address the traumas of his own childhood so as to be a more effective parent for Jane.

If the elephant in the room is simply the child's symptoms, as the drug companies would have us believe, then medication would appear to be the solution. Children taking medication for ADHD often tell me that it makes them feel calm. Risperidone, a powerful antipsychotic, undoubtedly can change a child's behavior. When it silences what the child is trying to communicate, making the true elephant in the room invisible, the full responsibility for the problem then falls squarely on the child's shoulders.

In another ironic link between the elephant advertisement and *God of Carnage*, one of the fathers in the play is an attorney representing a drug company. He speaks loudly on his cell phone, seemingly oblivious to the effect of his behavior on the other people in the room. The content of his conversation reveals the profit motive of the drug company taking precedence over the well-being of the patient.

God of Carnage contains an important message in a brief scene at the very end. The telephone rings and one of the mothers answers. It is her daughter, all upset about the loss of her pet hamster, which the father had "set free" one night because he was annoyed by the animal's habits. Suddenly the mood of the play, which was tense with barbed dialogue throughout, becomes serene as the mother speaks lovingly to her distraught daughter. Perhaps most of the audience was barely aware of the sudden mood change. Yet it gave this entertaining play a deeper significance. Freeing herself from the preceding chaos, she calmly gives her full attention to her daughter's experience.

The popularity of the play gives me hope that people are hungry for a different way to think about child and family troubles than the one offered by the pharmaceutical industry, which, with the money to place an attention-getting ad, has a very loud voice. It is joined by the equally loud voice of the private health insurance industry, which supports the quick fix of medication over more time-intensive treatments. In contrast, Mark, with his black smudge on my yellow wall, has a very small voice. His voice says, "Please think about my feelings, not just my behavior."

In School: The Untold Stories

High student/teacher ratios, lack of time for movement and free play, structured curricula, and testing all increase the pressure to diagnose psychiatric illness. For example, diagnosis of ADHD in children in low-income communities rose significantly in the wake of accountability to the No Child Left Behind act. In a school setting, teachers often must handle large groups of children, while having little training in working with kids from stressed family backgrounds who are struggling with emotional regulation. The pressure to control a disruptive child for the well-being of the whole class is understandable. When teachers have neither the time nor the backup to address underlying problems one-on-one, they may feel compelled to recommend an evaluation for medication, which can be effective in the short term.

With the advent of universal preschool, and a possible influx of children with problems of behavioral and emotional regulation, yet inadequate numbers of trained teachers and staff with space and time for listening, we run the risk of an exponential rise in prescribing of psychiatric medication. The 2011 change in the AAP (American Academy of Pediatrics) guidelines extending age of diagnosis of ADHD down from age six to age four (a move that was shortly followed by marketing of a new long-acting liquid form of ADHD medication) magnifies this risk.

A report from the Department of Education's Office of Civil Rights, highlighted in a *New York Times* editorial entitled "Giving Up on Four-Year-Olds," showed expulsion from preschool as a form of discipline occurring in increasing numbers. In one study, teachers were two and a half times more likely to expel, rather than suspend, a preschooler. Each child who is unable to function in preschool has a story. It takes time and a safe nonjudgmental environment to bring these stories to light and so make sense of a child's behavior. Often problems have been long standing, as we saw in Chapter 3, even dating back to infancy. Or behavior that makes it difficult for a child to tolerate the social structure of school may be related to frightening experiences, such as witnessing domestic violence at home. When a child lives in fear, she may respond to the "threat" of a child standing too close to her in line by pushing him. A reprimanding voice may lead to escalation of stress and even the development of a fight-or-flight reaction. Being sent to the principal's office can arouse fear and shame, leading already out-of-control behavior to escalate. Such a series of events might have preceded the recent incident of an eight-year-old boy, reportedly with a history of both trauma and ADHD, handcuffed by a law-enforcement official when teachers were unable to control his behavior.

In another common scenario, from the perspective of a child who is flooded and overwhelmed by a busy classroom, crawling under a desk may not be an indication of something wrong with her, but rather an adaptive response. Increasingly structured and crowded school environments, with little room to respond to the needs of an individual child, may exacerbate these problems.

Some innovative school programs around the country, informed by the ACE study that I describe in Chapter 4 and recognizing the effects of life experience on behavior, offer space and time for listening to the most vulnerable children. Jane Ellen Stevens writes about one such program—Lincoln High School in Walla Walla, Washington—on her blog *ACES Too High News*. In her post, the principal,

Jim Sporleder, describes how they respond to a child's problematic behavior not with punishment, but with listening. He offers an example of an interaction with a teen who exploded and cursed at a teacher. When Sporleder spoke quietly, noticing the intensity of his rage, the boy immediately reacted to this kindness—"The armor-plated defenses melt like ice under a blowtorch"—by talking about his alcoholic father who fails to keep promises. Sporleder explains that there were consequences to the student's behavior, but along with opportunity for healing. "He went to ISS—in-school suspension—a quiet, comforting room where he can talk about anything with the attending teacher, catch up on his homework, or just sit and think about how maybe he could do things differently next time."

James Redford, in his new documentary *Paper Tigers*, takes a close look at this program. In a blog post about his experience of doing the film, Redford writes: "I watched as teachers countered poor attitudes and poor choices by asking, "What's going on?" rather than "What's wrong with you?" The program has resulted in dramatic improvements in attendance, GPA, and graduation rates, with a parallel decrease in in-school fighting and school suspensions.

Given what we now know about the long-term effects of early childhood experiences, starting with the youngest children makes the most sense. At the Head Start–Trauma Smart Program at Crittendon Children's Center, in Kansas City, Missouri, three- to five-year-olds who come from environments of high stress are recognized as being physically and emotionally in "red alert" states. When behavior begins to unravel, they may be offered a "calm down box" and quiet time with a Trauma Smart therapist who can help them to regroup and regain emotional control. All those who interact with the children, including not only teachers and parents, but also bus drivers and cafeteria workers, receive training in trauma.

As psychiatrist Bessel Van der Kolk writes in his book *The Body Keeps Score*, "Children who defy the rules are unlikely to be brought to reason by verbal reprimands or even suspension—a practice that has become epidemic in American schools." Through the National Child Traumatic Stress Network he collaborates with schools to build a different model. Participating teachers' initial response is some version of "If I'd wanted to be a social worker, I'd have gone to social work school." But, he goes on, "teachers' perspectives begin to change when they realize that these kids' disturbing behaviors started out as frustrated attempts to communicate distress." These teachers, under guidance from Van der Kolk and his colleagues, learn to recognize and respond to these wordless communications. Rather than reprimanding or giving a time-out, they give words to a child's experience, using slow breathing and other techniques to help a child return to a calm state.

But these kinds of programs are the exception. And in schools everywhere, not only in identified "high-risk" populations, children struggle with similar issues. Teachers understandably prioritize keeping their classrooms safe. When faced with a disruptive child and a classroom of twenty to thirty children, without support from programs such as Van der Kolk's or embedded child development specialists, suspension or expulsion may feel like the only options.

The looming possibility of suspension or expulsion from school can put enormous pressure on parents. Pediatricians and psychiatrists often experience a flood of calls prior to the start of the school year, as parents panic about their child's ability to manage in the school setting. The expectation, for both parent and clinician, that they will leave the office with a prescription for medication is high.

"Medications Work, but Is That the Right Question?"

Whenever I raise these questions about psychiatric medication use in children, I receive an outpouring of comments from both the psychiatric community and parents whose children carry the ADHD label, that the medications help children to sit still and learn. While this may be true at first, there is evidence not only that these medications do not in the long term improve academic performance, but also that with current treatments the ADHD symptoms do not go away, and more serious mental illness, referred to as comorbidity, may emerge.

The very fact that psychiatric medications work so quickly and conveniently is part of the problem. The more effectively a medication eliminates symptoms, the more likely it will be used to silence children. Consider the extreme example of risperidone for a five-year-old for sleep. If such a study were ethically feasible, it is quite likely that risperidone would be found to be effective at getting young children to sleep. But the opportunity for growth and healing that accompanies discovering and treating the underlying cause of the problem, and for supporting development of healthy sleep patterns, would be lost.

The gold standard in ADHD treatment is the National Institute of Mental Health's MTA (Mulitmodal Treatment of ADHD) study, an $11 million study started over fifteen years ago. The study compared medication alone, behavior therapy alone, and a combination of the two. The results have engendered much controversy. While initially the study was used to tout the benefits of medication treatment alone, follow-up at three years failed to show any significant differences among the treatments. At the eight-year follow-up, many children still had symptoms of inattention and hyperactivity, even those who continued to take medication for the entire time. A long-term follow-up study of ADHD diagnosed in preschool showed similar results, with 90 percent of children continuing to experience symptoms six years after diagnosis and ongoing treatment with medication and/or behavior management.

Typical behavior management plans (sometimes referred to as behavior modification or behavior therapy) for treating ADHD involve targeting a specific problematic behavior, such as inattentive and distracted behavior while getting shoes on to leave the house for school. A motivational system, such as tokens or stickers, is applied in a consistent fashion to encourage the desired behavior. In the MTA study parents in the "behavior arm" received eight individual and twenty-seven group sessions to teach them behavior management techniques.

When we recognize behavior as communication, managing can be another form of silencing. As we have seen, battles over putting on shoes can have complex meaning. Lila described just this issue with her five-year-old daughter Hazel, referred to me for an ADHD evaluation. Efforts to leave the house often ended with Lila carrying her child, kicking and screaming, into the car. While Lila was eager to learn techniques to manage this behavior, I took a different approach. With a full hour available to us, Lila told me the following story while her infant son slept in his carrier.

She and her husband, Paul, had relocated to Boston from London for Paul's new job shortly before Hazel was born. Paul worked long hours and Lila's family was still living in London. The first year of Hazel's life was a lonely and isolated time for Lila. Now things had much improved. Paul was more involved with caring for both children and Lila had a large network of friends. However, as she told me this story, Lila seemed to connect with deep feelings of sadness as she thought of her own mother, and what she had lost by not having her close by when Hazel was an infant. While now she had a good support system, she still really missed her mother, especially as she was caring for a second baby. She recognized how Hazel's neediness provoked these feelings of loss. She easily became flooded with stress and was quick to anger. She said, "I wonder if Hazel feels like she's losing *me*." Hazel's increasingly oppositional and distracted behavior began to make sense, both to me and to her mother. It seemed that the two of them had become engaged in a dysfunctional dance of anger and provocative behavior. The fact that it occurred on the way out of the house, when Hazel would be in school and her mother home alone with the baby, likely aggravated the feelings of loss.

Following this visit, instead of yelling at Hazel to put on her shoes, Lila used praise and encouragement. Behind this change was not behavior management, but rather her insight into the meaning of Hazel's behavior. Hazel, in turn, sensing her mother thinking about her or "holding her in mind," willingly put on her shoes. Recognizing that Hazel's behavior was related to missing her, Lila offered Hazel some "special time" in the afternoon while the baby was sleeping. Hazel was rewarded, not with tokens or stickers, but by her mother's praise and attention and the calm that replaced the months of conflict.

If we had not taken the time to understand the meaning of this conflict, it is possible that, at least in the short term, her behavior would have improved with "management." However, if the feelings of sadness and anger disrupting the relationship between mother and daughter continued to go unacknowledged, the opportunity for healing might have been missed. The relationship might have deteriorated, leading to deeper and more complex emotional problems for Hazel.

Strikingly absent in the MTA study is opportunity to hear a family's story and wonder about the meaning of a child's behavior. Could it be that this lack of being heard, for both parent and child, is at the root of the poor long-term outcome? For clinicians under pressure to help in some way but without space and time to listen, the results indicating ineffectiveness of standard treatment may be hard to hear.

A defensive response may also occur when the long-term side effects of medication are questioned. A pediatrician colleague described difficulty getting a study published that explored the lack of research on the long-term safety of medications used to treat ADHD. The study from a group of physicians at Boston Children's Hospital concluded that "clinical trials conducted for [FDA] approval of many ADHD drugs have not been designed to assess rare adverse events or long-term safety and efficacy." The study was published in the open access online journal *PLOS ONE*. The authors first submitted the article to other widely read journals specifically for psychiatrists and pediatricians, but the article was rejected. According to the main author, "Reviewers were mainly concerned that we were being critical of ADHD drugs when they felt that there was a long-standing history of safety for many of these drugs." The study did not say anything about the drug's safety, but simply pointed out that studies that would answer this question did not exist. That this basic finding could not make its way into the journals that prescribers of these medications regularly read suggests a broad resistance among professionals who treat children with ADHD to ask these difficult questions.

When I made the decision, inspired by baby Haley, to devote my time to prevention, I was fortunate to have other options. My growing unease with the prescribing of psychiatric medication coincided with my discovery of the field of infant mental health. After giving the subject much careful thought, I decided to leave the ADHD practice that, as I described in Chapter 2, I'd inherited from a colleague. While I'd seen many children who have benefited in the short term from stimulant medication, I was troubled by the way medication is prescribed. The fact that the data does not demonstrate long-term benefits, and that the long-term side effects are open to question, added to my unease. I felt that I could no longer in good conscience prescribe stimulants year after year to large numbers of children. I could no longer stay silent and in doing so collude in this treatment. I wonder whether the defensive attitude I hear in my colleagues comes from the fact that in the current system of care, they do not see other options.

Seven

Prejudice Against Children

When I see young children silenced by labels and drugs in this way, I think of the work of Elisabeth Young-Bruehl, whose writing helped me like nothing else to understand how we as a society have gotten to this point.

Tragically, she died suddenly a month before the 2012 publication of her book *Childism: Confronting Prejudice Against Children*. Not only was this the loss of a great mind, but also the opportunity for her to represent her very important ideas, ones that would likely have caused continued controversy, in public discussion. An analyst, political theorist, and biographer, Young-Bruehl calls attention to the ways human rights of children are threatened. She defines *childism* as "a prejudice against children on the ground of a belief that they are property and can (or even should) be controlled, enslaved, or removed to serve adult needs."

Viewing a child's behavior as a "symptom" of a "disorder" that needs to be "managed" or eliminated with medication, rather than as a form of communication that needs to be heard, reflects this prejudice. It fails to recognize the child as a unique individual with his own thoughts, feelings, and needs. At the time of her death,

Young-Bruehl was in the process of editing Winnicott's complete works. His notion of the need to recognize a child's "true self" so as to encourage healthy development fits seamlessly with her ideas. My behavioral pediatrics practice again and again offers a microscopic view of the macroscopic trend Young-Bruehl so brilliantly articulates.

Defiance

Tears ran down Susan's cheeks as she described being so overwhelmed and full of rage that she forcefully held her fully clothed four-year-old son, James, under a cold shower when he wouldn't go to bed. Later in the same visit she revealed that she had suffered years of physical and emotional abuse as a child.

As is typical of visits to my practice, she had brought James because he was "defiant." "Something must be wrong with him" was followed by "Tell me what to do to make him behave." James's preschool teachers, who were having trouble managing his behavior, had suggested that he might have ADHD. They recommended to Susan that medication be considered. They knew nothing of her history.

I believe it was the expanse of time of the hour-long visit, together with my stance of nonjudgmental listening, that allowed Susan to tell me the full story so quickly. She must have been privately burdened not only by the knowledge of these frightening scenes, when both mother and child were helplessly out-of-control, but also by her recognition that she was repeating the trauma of her own childhood.

While Young-Bruehl does not write about the ADHD label, she writes of "a childism of the sort that is now fueling an epidemic of diagnoses of bipolar II disorder and the prescription of medications to children who are, in effect, being doped into acquiescence."

I wonder whether Young-Bruehl would find the use of the word *defiant* itself to be a manifestation of childism. Whole books are written about the defiant child, with such titles as *Your Defiant Child: 8 Steps to Better Behavior* by "ADHD expert" Russell Barkley. *Defiance* used in this way is a negative, judgmental word. Framing "defiant" behavior as a problem or even disorder, as in *oppositional defiant disorder*, or by the use of synonyms such as *disobedient* and *noncompliant*, is consistent with this view of children as property to be controlled. A colleague captured this sentiment in a powerful way when she said, "We need to stop feeling persecuted by our children." This term resonated for me, as that is exactly what parents convey when they describe their child's "challenging" or "impossible" behavior. One mother told me that she could talk on the phone only between three and three thirty, when her four-year-old daughter was napping. She felt that her daughter was controlling her, that she was powerless. In such a relationship, power struggles may replace understanding and connection.

When we have an opportunity to listen, we usually discover that "defiant" behavior actually represents a child's efforts to communicate his feelings. James's home felt unsafe and out of control. His behavior was not a sign of ADHD, but a cry for help.

"Defiant" behavior can push parents' buttons as nothing else. Following the release of my first book, I was asked to do an interview for a parenting blog about defiance. The interviewer also used the word *impudence*, another term with negative connotations. I suggested that this word projects intentions onto the child that are likely not his own. In fact, "defiant" behavior, when we explore the motivations from the child's perspective, grows out of an experience of not being understood.

Herein lies a possible explanation of why defiance pushes our buttons. In a sense, a parent is having exactly the same experience as the child. He is not being "seen" or recognized as an adult deserving of respect. A parent might have had other experiences of not being "seen," perhaps by a spouse, co-worker, or by his own parents, that makes him particularly vulnerable to getting upset about not being "seen" by his child.

In almost every instance of "defiant" behavior, if one digs a bit below the surface, the child's experience is not recognized. What we call "defiant" behavior usually represents a call for help because a child feels overwhelmed and defenseless. It might be that he is very sensitive to loud noises or taste, and battles around "making a scene" at a family outing or being a "picky eater" are related to these sensitivities. It might be a transient issue, such as his feelings being sidelined by a new baby, perhaps also with the effects of accompanying sleep deprivation. Or he may be absorbing the tension related to ongoing financial stress or marital conflict. Simply recognizing that these things are difficult for a child and acknowledging his experience, even if the stressors are still there, goes a long way in helping a child feel understood, and in turn decreasing "defiant" behavior.

A particularly dramatic example was the situation of six-year-old Maggie, who was brought to my practice with a chief complaint of "defiant" behavior. Further history revealed significant trauma in her life. An alcoholic father who had abandoned her as a toddler had recently been making visits, at which time he was often drunk and very loud. Yet her feelings about visits had not been discussed until they came to see me for behavior that was growing worse around bedtime. She refused to sleep in her own bed.

Once we had time to discuss this stressful situation, the need for her mother's company at bedtime for stories, comfort, and reassurance became clear. Maggie's mother saw that the father's intrusive behavior was as stressful for her daughter as it was for her, and when Maggie felt understood, her "defiant" behavior subsided.

While *defiant* usually has a negative meaning, it can also mean "bold." A dramatic example is the *Defiant Requiem*, a performance piece that has been made into a powerful film. It captures the World War II story of Jewish prisoners at the concentration camp Theresienstadt who, under the direction of fellow prisoner Rafael Schachter, using a single vocal score and legless piano, performed Verdi's *Requiem*. These performances offered a way to cling to life and dignity even as their ranks were repeatedly depleted with deportations to Auschwitz. This use of the word *defiant* represents a courageous assertion of the true self in the face of brutal silencing.

Limit Setting: The Time-Out Wars

Recent controversy around the use of time-outs calls attention to the way common discipline techniques are based in efforts to control behavior rather than support connection and communication.

For young children, limits on behavior are essential. Setting limits is a form of teaching, not controlling. Creating a containing environment, in which a child feels safe and able to handle big emotions, is a central role for parents. But how do we effectively set limits in a way that promotes healthy development? Psychiatrist Dan Siegel, father of the field known as interpersonal neurobiology, points to the shortcomings of this common discipline method. In a *Time* magazine piece, provocatively titled "Time-Outs Are Hurting Your Child," following the release of his new book *No-Drama Discipline*, he and colleague Tina Bryson wrote:

The problem is, children have a profound need for connection. Decades of research in attachment demonstrate that particularly in times of distress, we need to be near and be soothed by the people who care for us. But when children lose emotional control, parents often put them in their room or by themselves in the "naughty chair," meaning that in this moment of emotional distress they have to suffer alone.

Siegel advocates for "time-ins," whereby parents use a child's out-of-control feelings as an opportunity for teaching. Central to such an approach is for parents themselves to be able to name and control their own intense feelings. Discipline delivered in a state of rage defeats the purpose of both de-escalation and teaching of emotional regulation.

Lauren was sending her three-year-old son Oliver to his room for time-out multiple times a day. They were stuck in battles all day long. Lauren would tell Oliver, who as a typical example, wanted to watch TV before dinner, "If you ask again, you'll have to go to your room." Predictably, Oliver would ask again, descending into a screaming meltdown as his angry mother carried him kicking and thrashing to his room, where he was left alone. Lauren was mystified by the predictability of his response. "Why can't he just listen?" she asked.

Rather than focus on controlling Oliver's "oppositional" behavior, I offered Lauren and her husband, Ethan, a chance to tell the story from the beginning. As I find again and again, this simple process led them to a new way to understand what was happening. As both parents visibly relaxed, Lauren shed her defensive and angry stance. Ethan, who appeared haggard and anxious, looked hesitantly at his wife and then began to speak openly. He was worried about her emotional state. She easily lost her temper, screaming at Oliver or, when she felt she couldn't handle the situation, simply leaving him alone. While at first Lauren was uncertain about the relevance of her issues to Oliver's behavior, as she relaxed she admitted concern about the level of anger she felt. She had struggled with depression in the past, and since Oliver's birth the lack of regular sleep had affected her significantly. She knew that she needed to find ways to manage her feelings when Oliver's behavior provoked her. The stress of his mother's anger, and the isolation of time-out, had created a vicious cycle.

Once Lauren had time to think about this futile pattern of behavior she and her son had fallen into, and to wonder about what might be going on for Oliver, she was able to hear my ideas about helping Oliver in these out-of-control moments rather than leaving him alone. As we have seen repeatedly, Oliver's behavior could be reframed not as a problem to be managed but a form of communication, a way of saying, "I want to connect with you but I don't know how. I need your help with these big and difficult feelings."

The American Psychological Association annual meeting that followed the publication of Siegel's book included an entire symposium on the subject, titled "Children Need Positive Parenting and Timeout—A Rejoinder to the New Book *No-Drama Discipline*." Strikingly absent was any discussion of emotions; the focus was exclusively on behavior. If we recognize a child as an individual with thoughts and feelings of his own, and the way a child's behavior can push a parent's buttons, any discussion of appropriate discipline must include consideration of feelings, of both parent and child.

Dr. Siegel's main point is to not leave a child alone with out-of-control feelings. It is not the time-out per se, but rather the sense of abandonment that is potentially harmful. When a child is repeatedly abandoned both physically and emotionally in the middle of a meltdown, that experience in itself may be traumatic. He does not learn to manage his feelings. In such a situation frequency and intensity of meltdowns often worsens.

For young children, a matter-of-fact time-out in the face of biting or hitting can help teach them that this behavior is unacceptable. Even as young as eighteen months, most children can understand cause and effect, and will quickly learn when the process is consistent. Sitting in a specially designated spot (not their crib or room) can be more effective than verbal explanations that go beyond a child's understanding. Even for older children, in the midst of a meltdown they usually lose their thinking capacities, so gentle holding and a soft voice may be more effective than reasoning or explanations. Simply naming a child's feelings in these moments helps connect feelings with words, offering a sense of comfort and understanding. These forms of time-out do not involve physical or emotional abandonment.

But parents need to manage their own feelings first. I recommend finding ways to calm themselves in the heat of the moment, such as looking out a window and doing some deep breathing. Only then can parents help children recognize and contain their own big feelings.

A Societal Problem

Childism, as defined by Young-Bruehl, is a societal phenomenon. Individual parents, given the opportunity to be heard and supported, are not childist. They long to help their children, not merely control them. Susan, once she had the chance to tell her story of trauma, was eager to learn to regulate her emotions and help her son to manage his. She did not want to medicate away his symptoms. Nor are individual clinicians childist. They may feel themselves caught in a system of care that seems to offer few alternatives. For example, I have heard psychiatrists say that they have prescribed medication for a foster child in situations where, if behavior were not brought under control, the child would "lose his placement" and have another wrenching move to a different family. The preference, for professionals as well as families, is to find meaningful help, a space where a child can be heard and understood. Pediatricians, lacking time or training to handle the situation themselves, and facing severe shortages of mental health professionals for referrals, may be unable to provide further support and treatment. Not wanting to find a problem they cannot address, they may hesitate to uncover these underlying issues.

Young-Bruehl compares the situation in our country with that of comparably developed countries where "children have a range of preventative and development-oriented services: universal health care, health services, and parent support services in homes after the birth of a child; maternal and parental leaves for infant care; developmental preschool programs; after-school programs; and economic supports of various kinds." She astutely observes, "Children whose development is not being supported cannot be protected." She proposed a new Comprehensive Child Development Act to replace the one vetoed by Richard Nixon in 1972. I think she would be heartened by the recent policy statement of the American Academy of Pediatrics: "Early Childhood Adversity, Toxic Stress, and the Role of the Pediatrician: Translating Developmental Science into Lifelong Health." This policy statement seeks to use the explosion of research at the interface of neuroscience, genetics, and developmental psychology to support early parent-child relationships. It is a preventive model designed to promote healthy development.

But implementation of this policy will be difficult, if not impossible, unless space and time for listening is mandated and funded. Access to care is a significant obstacle. I believe Young-Bruehl would say that childism is the reason why professionals who work with children and families, including pediatricians, child therapists, and early childhood educators, are among the lowest paid. She would point to childism to explain why the health insurance industry and pharmaceutical industry have together been able to create a system where children are more likely to be medicated than listened to. She would say that medicating a child like James, or even using behavior management, without addressing either his mother's history of abuse or his experience of her out-of-control behavior would be a manifestation of childism.

Use of psychiatric medication for children in foster care offers a striking example of a societal prejudice against children. A powerful documentary film, *Drugging Our Kids*, an investigative series by the Bay Area News Group, documents this issue in a thorough and dramatic way, using interviews with young adults who were in the foster care system, some from as early as two years of age. They were labeled with multiple psychiatric diagnoses, when really what they were suffering from was trauma and loss. After experiencing physical, sexual, and emotional abuse, they were on multiple psychiatric medications for many years. With the help of a range of individuals who saw through the haze of drug effects to who they really were, those interviewed for the documentary were able to get off all medications. In a segment entitled "Treatment for a Broken Heart Is Not Another Medication," child psychiatrist David Arredondo says, "The first line treatment is not another medication. It is to understand, to listen to the child, to ask, 'what's going on, why are you sad in this way?'"

The film offers an even-handed approach, acknowledging that psychiatric medication can help children benefit from other forms of therapy, and in certain circumstances can be lifesaving. But, they point out, most often that is not the way these medications are used. Many children are on multiple powerful medications, with new ones added whenever there is an escalation in "problem behavior." Arredondo points to the fact that while we do not know the long-term effects of these medications on the developing brain, at the very least, large quantities of medication "blunt the developmental process."

Many of those interviewed for the documentary describe how psychiatric medications are used as "chemical restraints" to control a child's behavior. Angry, out-of-control behavior is a form of communication. It says, "I have never learned to manage my feelings. I have never been held in a loving and safe relationship." Medication silences that communication.

The children in the film have experienced trauma with a capital *T*. However, many children who are similarly diagnosed with psychiatric illness and medicated with psychiatric drugs have less dramatic trauma in their history. The Adverse Childhood Experiences (ACE) study I refer to in Chapters 4 and 6 offers extensive evidence that a range of adverse childhood experiences—including not only abuse and neglect, but also parental mental illness, separation and divorce, substance abuse, and domestic violence—are highly associated with both physical and mental health problems later on.

These cumulative experiences are a kind of trauma with a small *t*, more ubiquitous than frank physical and sexual abuse. The use of the word *trauma* itself can create a kind of "not me" reaction, while disturbing life events are actually quite common. Elegant and compelling research by Harvard psychiatrist Martin Teicher and colleagues found that in adults with diagnosed mental illness, the prevalence in childhood of what he terms "maltreatment," described as "repeated exposure to events that involve a betrayal of trust," is 42 percent. His research demonstrates that mental illness in the setting of a history of adverse childhood experiences is a very different entity, in terms of course of illness, response to stress, brain structure, and gene expression, than the same *DSM*-named disorders in the absence of these experiences. They show that it is meaningless to talk about mental health disorders, as defined by the *DSM* system, without knowledge of early life experience.

When we diagnose and medicate, without offering time and space for listening to stories, for healing through human connection, we are doing something quite similar to what was done to these foster care children, but in a more subtle and pervasive way. In contrast, when these stories are told and heard early, their effects on children acknowledged, and support offered for healing of troubled relationships, the opportunity for prevention is great.

Pediatrician T. Berry Brazelton, whose work is featured in Young-Bruehl's book as an antidote to childism, endorses her book, recommending that all who are involved with children and families should read it. Her book has helped me understand why it is so hard to get the kind of help for children that all the best science of our time is telling us they need. Young-Bruehl wisely recognizes that prejudice must be acknowledged in order to be overcome. I am hopeful that by taking a close up view of this subject, we will realize that protecting space and time for listening is not optional. It is imperative if we are to promote healthy growth and development of the next generation, and generations to come. In the following section I'll explore the kinds of listening, once the space and time is there, that best support this task.

Part Four

Ways of Listening

Eight

Listening to the Body: Paths to Healing

Sometimes it is the people no one imagines anything of who do the things that no one can imagine.

—*The Imitation Game*

Experiencing Calm

In the documentary *Drugging Our Kids*, DAnthony, one of the foster children interviewed, describes the role of music in his life. "Music keeps me out of trouble. I take anger and make music." Anna Johnson, a health policy analyst interviewed for the piece, speaks of the forms of self-expression, such as music, dance, and yoga, which help children to heal from trauma and connect with others who may have had similar experiences. "Music is about being better, being somebody." Out of dire circumstances, DAnthony uses music to discover his true self. When we can free ourselves from needing simply to control behavior, when we recognize behavior as communication, listening to that communication opens up a world of creative solutions, ways to calm both body and mind in the face of life's inevitable stresses.

When seven-year-old Adrian, who had been diagnosed with ADHD, was allowed to ride his scooter down the hall to his early-morning tutoring sessions, his attention and ability to take in information improved significantly. Helen, mom of three-year-old Asher, described the feeling of holding his body in the middle of a tantrum. His breathing would slow and his tense muscles relax as he melted into her lap. Then she remarked, it was as if his "thinking came back on line." Pediatrician T. Berry Brazelton, using the Neonatal Behavioral Assessment Scale, demonstrates how each newborn has a unique way of responding to light and sound. When a rattle is gently shaken near the ear of a sleeping baby, some babies will have a big response, with eyes squeezing closed and arms flying over their heads. Others, in contrast, will make some barely noticeable movement and then shut the sound out completely. Listening for the individual nature of a child includes listening to the body.

While this chapter focuses on listening to the child's body, it is equally important for parents to listen to their own body. To support healthy emotional development, they, too, need to feel calm and in control. When I ask a distraught parent, "Who takes care of you?" many offer a laugh and some variation of "I used to run, but I don't have time for that anymore." For many parents, the care of the body that allows for calm thinking goes out the window.

Listening to a child's communication requires a calm presence of mind, which may be unattainable if a parent has no time to care for herself. One mom, Brenna, asked me repeatedly to tell her what to do about her five-year-old daughter Amelia's tantrums. But she knew exactly what to do. In the quiet of my office, she could tell me in a calm, confident voice that she knew how to anticipate a meltdown and avoid it. She also knew that once Amelia had "lost it," she needed to be held and comforted until she could calm down. A third option, to put her in a brief time-out when she hit, would sometimes be needed. However, in the heat of the moment, rarely, if ever, did Brenna, whose husband worked twelve-hour days and often traveled for work, leaving her alone caring for four kids under the age of six, have the calm presence of mind to think clearly in this way.

A vivid example of employing self-regulation to manage a child's dysregulation is yoga for treatment of colic. By that, I mean yoga for Mom. As I grew to appreciate the role of the body in emotional regulation in my study of infant mental health, I saw the story of Nicole, Dan, and baby Haley from chapter three in a new light. I came to recognize just how significant Nicole's yoga class was in healing her relationship with her baby. At the time I attributed much of the transformation to having a chance to be heard both by me and by her husband. The yoga, too, had an important role to play.

My colleague Suzanne Zeedyk identifies the value of yoga in a blog post about a young mother whose children have been removed to foster care. Listening to her struggles to meet the parenting skills required by the child protection agency, Zeedyk wonders about the possibility of including a yoga class among all the required parenting classes. She points out that most mothers, like the one she writes about, have a history of trauma, but nothing is offered to support their own efforts at emotional regulation. She wisely observes that emotional regulation is perhaps the most important task not only for mothers in this extreme circumstance, but for mothers in many stressful situations. For example, when a baby has colic, or a mother is depressed, or both, this task of emotional regulation, of staying calm in the face of your child's distress, is very challenging. It is through self-regulation that a parent teaches this essential skill to a child. Zeedyk writes:

> In other words, children's brains and bodies can only learn what self-comfort and containment feel like when they have first experienced comfort and containment in the arms of a trusted adult. If the brain does not have the opportunity to know this state, then it will not build the synaptic connections that [enable] emotional regulation, later on in life. If a child does not have such neural pathways in place within the first few years of his/her life, then the battle to gain control of intense feelings may forever be a losing one.

Of course, yoga is not for everyone, and yoga classes are extraordinarily variable. The point is that parents need help with their own emotional regulation. Using the body to help the brain, through yoga, martial arts, swimming, or even simply walking can be an important intervention that is good for the whole family.

The "Orchid-Dandelion" Hypothesis

The "orchid-dandelion" hypothesis, described in a 2009 article in the *Atlantic* by David Dobbs, explores the genetic basis for the possibility of transforming vulnerabilities into adaptive assets. Behavioral genetics research has shown that there are genes associated with mental illness, but these genes are not necessarily expressed. The "orchid-dandelion" hypothesis proposes that these genes are associated with talents as well as vulnerabilities. The very sensitivities that make a person at risk for mental illness in an unsupportive environment can lead to achievement and success in a supportive environment.

Offering evidence to support this theory, researchers in Melbourne, Australia, recently identified a gene that raises the odds of depression in people who have suffered abuse. But individuals with the very same gene, in the absence of such trauma, tend to be happier than people who do not have the gene variant. In a press release, the lead author described the significance of his findings: "This research tells us that what may be considered a risk gene in one context, may actually be beneficial in another."

In a beautiful example of transforming a vulnerability into an asset, Philip Schultz, now a Pulitzer Prize–winning poet, describes in his book *My Dyslexia* how he struggled terribly as a child with what is today recognized as dyslexia. While the subject of learning disabilities is beyond the scope of this book, his story offers an example of turning a challenge into a strength. Schultz describes how his mother would read his favorite comics over and over again with the hope that this would help him make sense of words. This kind of tolerance and patience gave Schultz the space to invent a new way of reading that was adapted to his particular form of dyslexia.

Schultz describes not only his academic struggles, but also how he was kicked out of one school for hitting other children when they called him "stupid." I wonder whether, had he been a child today, he might have been described as "impulsive" and "distracted," classic symptoms of ADHD. Had his symptoms been medicated away, he might not have invented his new way of reading, a method he now uses to teach others with similar difficulties to write fiction and poetry. He might not have become a poet, much less win the Pulitzer Prize.

As another example, while at preschool Michelle, a sensitive child, would often put her hands over her ears and run in circles, overwhelmed by the level of activity in school. She did not engage in play with other children. An experienced teacher suggested she be evaluated for possible autism spectrum disorder. A psychiatrist specializing in the disorder confirmed this suspicion and recommended further evaluation.

Her parents, noticing her extreme sensitivity to a range of sensory experiences, took a different approach. They made efforts to anticipate the kinds of experiences that set her off. With her verbal abilities lagging behind, she could not express herself and simply acted out in the face of sensory overload. Sometimes this involved running around in circles at preschool, rather than joining the group. Sometimes it was loud screaming, kicking, and thrashing when she had to leave a place or activity she was enjoying. They made a conscious effort to expose her to the world in a way that she could tolerate.

Michelle is now a talented musician and honors student. Her home is often filled with friends playing music together. In stark contrast to that little girl who exploded at the slightest provocation, she is a calm, quiet, thoughtful teenager.

Michelle is an example of an "orchid." In her early years, her behaviors might easily have been labeled as some type of disorder. Stressful life events and lack of an attuned environment might have put her at risk for significant mental health problems. But her parents resisted the pressure to label her; instead listening patiently and helping her navigate challenging situations.

As she had the opportunity to grow and develop, these "problems" of early childhood were transformed into talents. Her sensitivities, which made it difficult for her to form friendships when she was young, were the very qualities that led her to deeper and meaningful friendships as she grew into adolescence.

Sensory Differences

Sensitivities such as those exhibited by Michelle often lie behind a range of behavior problems. A child for whom sights, sounds, and touch are intense and overwhelming may develop rituals to help her manage the disorganizing effect of this experience. Challenges of picky eating may have their roots in intense responses to taste. Difficulty managing personal space may be linked with variations in proprioception, or sensing the position of the body. These behaviors may earn children the label of obsessive-compulsive disorder (OCD) as well as possibly ADHD, anxiety disorder, or autism. Similar behavior traits and diagnoses are often present in many other family members.

Winnicott anticipated our current knowledge of the role of sensory processing in emotional development. Of the "holding environment" that offers both understanding and security, he writes:

> [It] takes account of the infant's skin sensitivity-touch, temperature, auditory sensitivity, visual sensitivity, sensitivity to falling (action of gravity) and the infant's lack of knowledge of anything other than itself.

Controversy swirls around the question of whether "sensory integration disorder" should be included in the DSM system. The use of the word *disorder* may have the effect of diverting our attention from addressing the issues in a meaningful way. A diagnostic label may be required by the health-care system in order to get services covered by insurance. But the need to find something "wrong" with a child may get in the way of giving her time to become aware of her sensitivities and learn to tolerate and manage them. Rather than asking, "Is it a disorder?" but instead, "What is her experience of the world, and how can we help her make sense of and manage that experience?" we incorporate the child's unique sensory profile into understanding the meaning of her behavior.

Sensory processing differences may appear as a "problem" in some environments and not others. A middle child with sensitivity to sounds who has loud, boisterous siblings may struggle, whereas an only child whose parents can easily accommodate her needs may thrive. Or differences may be more pronounced as a result of a developmental issue—as in a child with delayed language development who cannot effectively communicate her physical aversion to intense flavors. By taking time to recognize an individual child's unique circumstances, both parents and professionals can help a child incorporate these traits into her emerging sense of self in a positive way.

Finding support for parents is equally important. Caring for a child like Michelle may engender feelings of inadequacy, self-doubt, and helplessness in parents. Integrating a child's vulnerabilities into the day-to-day realities of life in a hectic household can be a constant challenge. Validating these experiences, and recognizing their effects on the family dynamic, including relationships between parents and among siblings, can help prevent these issues from exerting negative effects on family functioning.

Thinking About Feelings

Kim and Jason came to me at their wits' end over four-year-old Jonathan's frequent meltdowns. "He's been like this from birth," said

Kim at our first visit. She described needing to nurse Jonathan as an infant in a dark, quiet room because he was so easily distracted by sights and sounds. When I asked them to tell me about a recent specific moment of disruption, they described a visit to a county fair, where, despite the abundance of appealing snacks, when he was clearly so hungry that he was falling apart, he refused to eat. Kim had lost her cool, yelling at him in the face of what seemed like irrational behavior. Finally, recognizing the futility of this battle, they gave up and took him on a hayride. At the conclusion of the ride, to the astonishment of his beleaguered and exhausted parents, he asked for a hot dog, as if nothing had happened. "In a sense, he's still that infant you nursed in that quiet, dark room," I said. Both nodded in agreement and recognition.

When we took the time to look at the moment in detail, by slowing things down, it was very clear that the intense stimulation of the fair overwhelmed him, and only with the gentle movement of the hayride, when his body could again feel calm and organized, could he focus on eating.

Next, Kim went on to describe a difficult visit to a butterfly museum, where, as she demonstrated, he winced and withdrew his entire body when a butterfly came near him. He was trapped between fear and desire, as he longed to be like the other kids and have one land on his shirt. He became increasingly frustrated, and finally disrupted the whole outing. For Kim, the day had been a humiliating failure that she just wanted to forget. But now, in this safe environment when she could stand to take a closer look, the significance of his sensory experience was vividly clear.

When I next saw the family, Kim described an apple-picking adventure. This time they let him ride the tractor rather than insisting they first pick apples. They saw how the movement calmed him. The rest of the outing was a success. Kim and Jason helped

Jonathan notice that he had a hard time calming down when there was a lot going on, and that movement helped him feel settled. Over time, as his parents gave words to his experience and he grew to understand his vulnerabilities, he learned how to calm himself in the face of overstimulation.

Child psychiatrist Stanley Greenspan called attention to the way in which a child's sensory experience of the world is closely connected with her ability to manage intense emotions. When caregivers help a child to recognize this connection, they help her become a reflective thinker, with an ability to think about feelings, and in doing so, learn to regulate them. Reflective thinking is intimately tied with emotional regulation and social adaptation. Naming the child's adaptive attempt to protect herself from sensory overload as a disorder, and eliminating disruptive behavior without exploring its meaning, leads to missed opportunities for developing these abilities that are central to overall mental health.

Greenspan suggested that many DSM-defined disorders, including ADHD, are problems of emotional regulation and sensory processing. He developed a model of assessment and intervention for young children with a range of developmental and behavioral challenges he termed DIR™. "D" for Developmental refers to the idea that to understand and treat children with a variety of behavioral difficulties, it is essential to understand the child's level of development. The "I" refers to Individual differences, as described on his website as "the unique biologically-based ways each child takes in, regulates, responds to, and comprehends sensations such as sound, touch, and the planning and sequencing of actions and ideas." He emphasizes the need to capture each child's unique sensory processing profile. The "R" refers to the way in which development and individual differences evolve within the context of

Relationships. DIR Floortime™ is a form of treatment whose effectiveness in treating a range of problems has been documented by extensive research. Similar to Winnicott's play space, Floortime™ offers time and space to recognize a child's unique circumstances and to listen to parent and child together.

A recent policy statement from the American Academy of Pediatrics on the role of sensory integration therapies for children with developmental and behavioral disorders cautions against using the diagnosis of "sensory processing disorder," claiming that sensory integration problems are likely to be symptoms of some other disorder, such as autism or anxiety. As with an Escher print, however, this interpretation may depend on how the situation is viewed. As we learn more about the underlying genetics and neuroscience, we may find instead that the sensory processing issue is primary. In the *DSM* system we are simply categorizing the range of behavior that results from this experience into diagnoses, such as autism, OCD, anxiety, and depression.

As Greenspan identified, our sensory experience is intimately tied to our ability to manage ourselves in a complex social environment. The world may feel soft and inviting, or harsh and dangerous. Consider this poignant description from Daphne Merkin, in a *New York Times Magazine* piece about her lifelong struggle with depression: "It is an affliction that often starts young and goes unheeded—younger than would seem possible, as if in exiting the womb I was enveloped in a gray and itchy wool blanket instead of a soft, pastel-colored bunting."

Many of the children I have seen over the years who were "explosive," or "inflexible," or challenging in other ways as young children, were also easily overwhelmed by a variety of sensory experiences.

One little boy I saw in my behavioral pediatrics practice carried a diagnosis of selective mutism. While he talked freely in every other setting, he refused to speak in school. He was eventually able to tell his parents that he experienced colors as sounds. This is a variation of sensory processing known as synesthesia, where two sensations are combined. For example, sounds are experienced as having color. Certainly it alters a child's perception of the world. For this boy, the new stimulation in the classroom was overwhelming. These qualities may be associated with great talents, particularly musical. Until he found the words to express and make sense of his experience, he protected himself with silence. Young children with similar sensory sensitivities may become very distracted in the school setting and receive a diagnosis of ADHD. Again, the sensory issue may be primary, and the behavior labeled "ADHD" secondary.

An occupational therapist trained in principles of infant mental health will recognize the relational nature of sensory problems and work with parent and child together. I have heard parents describe certain kinds of occupational therapy that, leaving parents in the waiting room, included listening to tapes to "reprogram" a child's brain. Yet if parent and child are separated in this way, the meaning of a symptom within the context of relationships may not be discovered. While sensory integration differences may originate in the child, her experience immediately takes on meaning within relationships.

A newborn who is not cuddly and does not like to be held may evoke feelings of shame and even depression in a mother. A father who himself had sensory processing challenges but experienced verbal humiliation or a slap across the face because of his difficulties may be overwhelmed with anxiety, paralyzed in the face of his child's similar struggles. Sibling relationships may be significantly affected as parents' attention is diverted to support the needs of a more vulnerable child. When one parent, having had these same struggles as a child, identifies with the child's experience, that parent may be more understanding. In this situation the other parent may blame that parent, not only for passing these traits on to the child, but also for being "indulgent." With time to listen and reflect there is opportunity to unwrap all the multiple variations and complexities these sensory sensitivities engender in families.

Using the Body to Help the Brain

The rush to diagnose, manage, and medicate may lead us to miss opportunities to use movement to support healthy brain growth and functioning. The Neurosequential Model of Therapeutics that I refer to in Chapter 4 is based on knowledge of brain development. Dr. Perry's model focuses on the fact that in order to think, learn, and process experience, one must first feel calm. The lower "feeling" centers of the brain need to be engaged before the higher "thinking" centers can work properly. Perry's ideas grew out of his frustration with the traditional model of psychiatric care, where children who have experienced significant trauma, treated only with medication, are expected to sit and talk with a therapist about their experience in weekly therapy. He recognized that this approach was failing.

He introduced us to his model during the Infant-Parent Mental Health program that I refer to in Chapter 3, speaking to our group about the importance of what he referred to as "rapid alternating movements" in achieving emotional regulation. Before a child can begin to talk about difficult experiences, the higher thinking centers need to be working. In times of stress, such as being reprimanded in a loud and busy classroom, a child may have use of only the lowest centers of her brain that control basic regulatory functions, such as breathing and heart rate. The higher centers that control emotion and thinking may in a sense go "offline." A child may have no sense of time other than of that moment. Traditional approaches of punishment, along with well-intentioned explanations of appropriate behavior, will not be effective when the thinking parts of the brain are not working. Parents who try to reason with a child in the middle of a tantrum know this all too well.

The common experience of taking a walk to cool down is an example of using rapid alternating movements to help the lower centers of the brain function more evenly, in a better-regulated fashion. Being outside, particularly in nature, may itself have a regulating and calming effect. A range of activities can achieve this calm. Dr. Perry does therapy sessions with very troubled children while going on walks. Horseback riding, martial arts, drumming, and dance are other activities that serve to organize, calm, and regulate the brain. When the brain is regulated, so are emotions, thinking, and behavior. A group of us in the Infant-Parent Mental Health Program got to try out the theory. After a long, very stimulating (and also somewhat overwhelming) day of learning with Dr. Perry, we went ice-skating. Not only was it a lot of fun, but it also worked wonders in helping us process what we had learned and make sense of it.

Often when kids struggle in school, teachers express concern that with arts and sports programs they are "overscheduled." But when we recognize the central role of these activities in thinking and learning, we see that they are not "extra." If such activities are carefully planned and well thought out, they add essential support to learning and healthy development. Ideally this approach involves interspersing some kind of a calming activity between sessions of homework, tutoring, or therapy. These can be tailored to a child's particular talents and interests.

Several years after his wise tutor discovered the scooter as a teaching tool, Adrian had learned to recognize that when he was feeling overwhelmed, going down to the basement to play his drums helped him regroup. This kind of awareness, both of mind and body, can serve kids well not only in childhood, but also over the course of a lifetime as they learn to adapt to their particular vulnerabilities.

Another advantage of activities, such as martial arts, horseback riding, and swimming is that they involve intimate relationships with teammates, coaches, and instructors. Many martial arts instructors offer classes for parent and child together. Both the relationship and the body help grow and heal the brain. It is not simply the physical activity, but the empathic connections formed and the sensitive listening that occurs in the context of these activities.

Recent research exploring the role of exercise in treatment of ADHD points to a broadening in our understanding of problems in regulating emotion, behavior, and attention. In one study, children diagnosed with ADHD were found to have better thinking skills when they engaged in intense physical activity. In a widely read article published in the *Washington Post*, a pediatric occupational therapist suggests a link between the lack of all kinds of movement in school and the rise in ADHD diagnoses. Standing desks, increasingly being used in classrooms, offer one adaptation to a child's need to move so as to think well.

Listening to the body of an individual child means giving consideration, based on that child's strengths and vulnerabilities, to what kind of physical activity is helpful, how and when it occurs, and whether it occurs in the context of meaningful relationships. In fact, for a young child who is overwhelmed by sensory experience, as are many children diagnosed with ADHD, traditional gym may precipitate an increase in disorganization and hyperactivity.

Infant massage, a well-known tool for supporting early parent-infant relationships, offers another example of using the body to help the brain. At a recent ICDL (Interdisciplinary Council on Development and Learning) conference, an organization founded on the ideas of Stanley Greenspan, I learned about a program, "Nurturing Touch: Infant and Pediatric Massage," in Montclair, New Jersey, where therapists do massage with drug-addicted moms and their babies who are being treated for withdrawal symptoms. The woman who described the program explained that at first she just worked with the babies, and held what she soon recognized were incorrect assumptions about the mothers. She observed, "We rip the mothers and babies apart" when there is a positive toxicology screen (drugs found in the urine). When she actually met the mothers, she found that they were in deep pain over being separated from their babies and longed to reconnect with them. She began to use her massage techniques on the mothers as well, recognizing that many of them had histories of abuse, and might never have experienced touch in a positive and caring way. She did this simply with gentle hand massage. Her aim was to begin to relax their bodies enough to enable them to hold their own very dysregulated babies, providing comfort both mother and baby so desperately needed. Offering these kinds of interventions for stressed mother-baby pairs, examples of using the body to help the brain in early development, may go a long way in preventing more complex problems of sensory and affective experience.

Creativity in Healing

A number of years ago I discovered the work of Vered, a musician and music therapist, when she reached out to me by e-mail. She began studying clinical psychology after the birth of her first child.

But rather than complete her PhD, she produced an album for parents and babies, *Good Morning My Love*, which won the Parents' Choice Gold Award. I found the following on her website:

> The benefits of music are intuitive. . . . Music, with its inherent melody, rhythm, and repetition, is a language that babies can understand from day one. It also has a way of organizing experience and enhancing it. Both you and your baby can use music to create routine, develop reliable patterns of expectations, and foster a sense of security—all of which help create a familiar and loving environment.

As a lover of folk music, I was captivated. One song that is excerpted on her website perfectly captures the ambivalence of toddlerhood, with the lyrics, "Mama leave me be but don't leave me." In groups for moms and babies, she uses music to address the anxiety and isolation that new moms often feel.

The therapeutic value of music became clear in my work with five-year-old Maddie, who struggled with severe social anxiety. The lunchroom and gym were particularly difficult, and she would retreat into silence. In a visit with her parents, we were discussing how to approach the teachers about making her comfortable in school. We had a full-hour appointment with plenty of time to hear her parents' story. That's when her father observed, "You know, she loves classical music." Her mother described a recent family gathering where there had been a lot going on and Maddie was quite agitated. But when someone put on some classical music, she became completely calm and seemed at peace.

We began to brainstorm about how they might make use of this observation in the school setting. For some reason she couldn't process all the sensory information coming at her in a busy social scene. But with the help of classical music, it was as if the neurons, the cells of her brain, lined up and began to work properly.

This visit got me thinking about a movie, *The Music Never Stopped*, based on the story of an actual patient as described by neurologist and writer Oliver Sacks in his essay "The Last Hippie." The movie's main character is a young man who suffered severe brain injury and was socially disconnected even from his immediate family. Before the injury he had been a passionate musician. His family, with the help of a music therapist, discovered that when he listened to the music from before his injury, he became completely clear-thinking and engaged. Like my young patient, his brain was a place of confusion and disorganization until the music allowed things to, in a sense, fall into place.

Kayla's story provides a beautiful example of an innovative approach to healing. Kayla was first brought to me in a whirlwind of panic on the part of family members, doctors, and teachers. There was great pressure, both on her mother, Jessica, and on me, to diagnose a disorder and to medicate her. She was only 4 years old. She had been adopted at three months after living with a drug-addicted mother. She had experienced many losses. Because of Kayla's hyperactive behavior and erratic sleep patterns, no one in the house had slept well for months. As we had a full hour for each visit, I was able to expand our conversation—to learn about family relationships and other ongoing stressors, including the recent separation of Kayla's parents. Sometimes I met with Jessica alone, offering her the opportunity to explore these difficult subjects openly. At other times, Kayla came too—visits that at first felt chaotic. But with time Kayla began to connect and play in an organized way. After we had met once a month for about six months, the whole situation had calmed down significantly. She was sleeping through the night and was listening in school and beginning to make friends.

One day as we sat on the floor in a moment of quiet, while Kayla sat at the small table drawing, Jessica said, "We discovered she loves to knit." When I expressed surprise that a child this young could knit, Jessica shared her story. When Kayla was an infant, Jessica would often knit beside her crib. As soon as Kayla was old enough to walk, she climbed out of her crib one day, and taking her mother's knitting needles from the table, began to tap them against each other. Jessica wondered whether she associated the gentle rhythmic sound with their peaceful quiet times together. As Kayla grew she learned to create the same sound and rhythm, enjoying the activity and soothing herself at the same time.

With this telling of her knitting story, Jessica saw how it was helpful not only to Kayla, but also in reconnecting with her own mother. Jessica's relationship with her mother had been fraught for years. They often fought over how to "manage" Kayla. But they, too, shared this love of knitting. Perhaps, Jessica wondered, the knitting connected Kayla with her in the same way it connected her with her own mother. Following this visit, Jessica recognized that she could make use of the knitting in a more purposeful way. The three generations began to have daily knitting sessions—a kind of family knitting club that offered peaceful calm, connection, and healing.

Coming up with such unique solutions requires an expanse of time. In contrast, lack of time for listening, with the rush to find a quick answer, closes off this opportunity. Knitting and music can be part of growth and healing that match a specific set of issues in an individual child and family. Time and space gives us opportunity to notice significant things that we might otherwise overlook. The feeling of safety and the freedom to wonder help parents discover ways to support and develop their child's strengths.

Theater and Storytelling

In his book *The Body Keeps Score*, psychiatrist and trauma researcher Bessel Van der Kolk offers a comprehensive overview of our knowledge of how stress lives in the body, and how using the body can help a person to heal from extreme stress or trauma. An innovative theater program in Lenox, Massachusetts, "Shakespeare in the Courts," offers an example. Van der Kolk describes how "[teenagers] found guilty of fighting, drinking, stealing, and property crimes, are sentenced to six weeks, four afternoons a week, of intensive acting study." This experience gives vulnerable children an opportunity to give words to their feelings, an important step on the road to emotional regulation. Many who come from disrupted home environments may not have developed the capacity for reflective thinking. One result is the impulsive behavior, literally acting without thinking, which got them in trouble. Van der Kolk describes how the director Kevin Coleman draws out this kind of reflection. Rather than asking, "How did it feel?" which invites judgment, "Coleman asks, 'Did you notice any specific feelings that came up for you in that scene?' That way they learn to name emotional experiences . . . The more they notice, the more curious they get." In a sense, the theater program supports the teenagers' ability to listen to themselves, to find meaning in their own behavior.

Van der Kolk quotes Tina Packer, founder of Shakespeare and Company, sponsor of the program: "Therapy and theater are intuition at work . . . What makes therapy effective is deep subjective resonance and that deep sense of truth and veracity that lives in the body." Reaching that "deep sense" is very like Winnicott's notion of connecting with one's true self.

In another example, at our local elementary school, a theater program is in full swing by third grade. Many young children who struggle in a variety of ways make wonderful use of this opportunity. I will never forget one young girl, diagnosed with Tourette's syndrome, with a significant stutter, who at the age of ten in a lead role sang with powerful force and clarity, with no trace of her disability onstage. I have seen many children over the years not only grow into themselves, but also discover remarkable talents that influence the course of their development through high school and beyond.

Theater is a form of storytelling. Storytelling allows for finding meaning in behavior. In the afterword of his book about the annual creativity seminar at the Austen Riggs Center, psychologist M. Gerard Fromm writes, "The Austen Riggs Center, which is home to . . . the Creativity Seminar, can be seen as an archive of the stories that need to be told but were not able to be heard, and because not able to be heard, could not be told—except in symptoms, nightmares and actions. From this angle, psychopathology is suppressed creativity and psychological growth is about storytelling and story listening."

When we have time to listen, we can offer a safe space for expressing feelings of pain and sadness that are inevitably part of the story. The following chapter will show how the process of mourning is central to growth and healing.

Nine

Listening for Loss: Time and Space for Mourning

Touch it; the marble eyelids are not wet:
If it could weep, it could arise and go.

—Elizabeth Barrett Browning,
Grief

Give sorrow words; the grief that does not speak knits
up the o'er wrought heart and bids it break.

—William Shakespeare,
Macbeth

In his book *The Examined Life*, psychoanalyst Stephen Grosz tells
why he includes Charles Dickens's *A Christmas Carol* on a reading list for a course on psychotherapy. Scrooge's transformation
over the course of visits from the three ghosts, he explains, offers
an example of how people change. He writes:

But Dickens' tale points to a further, darker and unexpected truth. Sometimes change comes not because we set out to fix ourselves, or repair our relation to the living; sometimes we change most when we repair our relations to the lost, the forgotten, the dead. As Scrooge grieves for those he had loved but put out of his mind, he begins to regain the world he had lost. He comes to life.

A number of years ago I was using another pediatrician's office while developing a new program focused on emotional health in families with children under age five. While I had brought toys, pens, and paper, I kept forgetting the tissues. Parents who cried would sniff and wipe their nose on sleeves, while I looked on, not wanting to disrupt the experience by running out of the room for supplies. Finally I remembered. In my practice I increasingly recognized the importance of expressing feelings of sadness, of moving through emotional pain on the road to healing.

Carol, a young mom who could shift rapidly from easy humor to overwhelmed anxiety, sat tensely at the edge of her seat, imploring me to tell her what to do about her five-year-old daughter Charlotte's refusal to eat "real food." They engaged in multiple daily battles, with Charlotte's food choices becoming increasingly narrow. Carol spoke quickly and urgently, with the pressured, insistent nature of her speech making the task of finding meaning a challenge. But I knew that if I simply told her what to do, as many others, including her pediatrician, already had, we would all fail. Information about her child's natural appetite, about letting her make her own choices, was not getting through. Something was in the way. And none of us knew what it was.

In an effort to connect with the feelings behind her words and behavior, I commented that she loved her daughter so much and was so worried about her. This comment opened a break in the armor. As her voice cracked, even as she continued to insist that I tell her what to do, I noticed her reaction. "What did I say that affected you?" I asked. Then came the flood of tears. At first she tried to fight the feeling, contorting her face in an effort to maintain her usual good humor. But as I sat quietly, she seemed to relax into her sadness, letting the tears flow freely. She spoke of being terrified of "screwing up" her daughter. She described a painfully fraught relationship with her own mother, in the face of numerous food aversions that persisted from childhood through her adult life.

Carol identified so closely with her young daughter that she couldn't believe in the child's natural ability to read her body's hunger signals. Carol felt herself fused with her daughter, unable to separate her own experience. The issue of eating had become intimately intertwined with the developmental task of separation.

We were able to find our way to this meaning only when Carol had space and time to connect with her sadness over her relationship with her own mother. Not that we had fully addressed this problem, as Carol might choose to do in her own therapy, but we had identified the way these painful feelings were affecting her experience as a parent, having landed on this fraught subject of eating. Only then could she move these feelings out of the way and hear the advice about letting Charlotte make her own choices. At a subsequent visit, Carol shared the fruits of our labor in a delightful story. Still in the grips of her anxiety, she had asked Charlotte why she would eat strawberries for her aunt but not for her mother. Charlotte had replied clearly and emphatically, "I ate the strawberries for me."

Giving advice, as well as parent training and behavior management, sometimes collectively referred to as psychoeducation, are left-brain, thinking activities. To change the way we behave, we need to change the way we feel. Giving space and time for mourning, when the right-brain, or feeling, centers can be activated, encourages this kind of change. Carol came to the visit with a wish for me to tell her what to do. But she agreed, after this wave of deep sadness had a chance to wash over her and then pass, that she had known for some time what to do. She just couldn't do it. Her fears about harming Charlotte, intimately intertwined with her grief about her relationship with her mother, were in the way. In expressing feelings of sadness over her own loss, she could see her daughter as a separate person. In this sense, mourning can lead to recognizing a child's true self.

Pixar's clever and profound film *Inside Out*, by making emotions into actual characters, highlights their essential contribution in guiding our thinking, perception, and social interactions. But perhaps most importantly, the film gives a starring role to the character of blue, round, bespectacled Sadness in moving through loss to healing, growth, and joy.

It is not simply that crying makes a person feel better. Hidden behind a child's "problem behavior" is often a story of loss, not only of death, but also of relationships that are unhealed. Those old wounds may be in the way of seeing children as themselves. While healing those relationships may be a separate and more long-term endeavor, naming them and experiencing them in real time can help parents think about their children's feelings. When there is no safe space to let go of the intense sadness, warding off grief may be a healthy adaptation. But these still raw feelings of loss may get in the way of the empathy and full presence that supports healthy development. Once parents are able to put such feelings in their rightful place, the behavior problem is more likely to resolve.

A number of years ago I attended a workshop at Austen Riggs entitled "The Interplay of Psychoanalysis and Buddhism." While

I did not know very much about Buddhism, having been greatly influenced by psychoanalysts D. W. Winnicott and Peter Fonagy, I was curious to learn more about this relationship. In particular I was interested in the place of mourning in Buddhism, for I had increasingly come to recognize that meaningful change, and with it the joy of connection, often occur when parents move through moments of profound sadness.

Workshop leader Joseph Bobrow's kind, gentle manner conveyed a sense of quiet authority that was calming and containing. He described the Buddhist notion of "reauthoring our suffering." He described how sadness can "hijack us," but that how by telling our story in a nonjudgmental environment, out from under the shadow of shame, the story can "take its place in a hierarchy." He described tolerating the sadness, letting it happen with the hope that the sorrow can then be transformed into one of the "waves of life." He spoke of how the therapist's "presence of mind" makes this possible, offering that calm, regulation, and healing.

As Bobrow spoke about meditation and Zen Buddhism, I was struck by the idea of meditation as a process of noticing how we become derailed by patterns of thought and behavior. I thought about how in my own work, when I help parents to slow things down, they become aware of how their child's behavior provokes them, and how they may unintentionally attribute meaning to their child's behavior that is markedly different from the child's true intention.

When I help a parent to move from "he never listens" or even "he's terrible" to instead describing a very specific moment of disruption in great detail, he may suddenly see how his child's behavior provokes his own memories of loss and feelings of grief. One father recognized in his response to his daughter's "defiance" a surge of rage that he linked to a memory of his own father's slapping him across the face. A mother shifted from anger at her husband's lack of support with her son's meltdowns to profound pain over the gradual erosion of her failing marriage. Bobrow seemed to put this shift into words as he described an opportunity to "use the suffering to turn straw into gold." For in the face of this realization, of this "riding the wave" of sorrow, these parents could "reauthor the suffering" and in doing so separate their own experience from that of their children.

When these deep feelings of sadness are buried and unexpressed, they can wreak havoc on current relationships. In contrast, when parents are aware of the feelings a child provokes, and given opportunity to mourn these losses in a safe, containing environment, they can move them off the child. As they slow down, parents begin to see the child as himself. In turn, the child, himself feeling recognized and understood, becomes calm. This meditative process can be what leads to the moments of profound joy and connection between parent and child that follow.

Loss as Part of Parenting

When we become parents, we have the opportunity to open our hearts to a love unlike any other. But in opening ourselves to this love, we become vulnerable to loss. Loss is an inevitable part of parenting. That simple step of putting a baby to bed for the first time in his own room is full of poignancy. It is the first of many losses as our children grow up. The first day of kindergarten, going off to college, and all the many small steps toward becoming a separate, independent individual are mixed with ambivalence and loss for both parent and child. And though the idea is mostly out of our conscious awareness, in becoming parents we make ourselves vulnerable to an unlikely but real possibility of unbearable loss.

A central task of parenting is to manage our anxiety around loss. Not only when we put our children to bed, but when we let them go down a slide, go to preschool, or go skiing in the mountains. We allow them to separate and grow up. All along we must learn to manage our deep, complex feelings of sadness and worry.

I recently came upon a beautiful, if exquisitely painful, expression of this idea in Hanya Yanagihara's novel A *Little Life.*

You have never known fear until you have a child, and maybe that is what tricks us into thinking it is more magnificent, because the fear itself is more magnificent. Every day, your first thought is not "I love him" but "How is he?" The world, overnight, rearranges itself into an obstacle course of terrors. I would hold him in my arms and wait to cross the street and would think how absurd it was that my child, that any child, could expect to survive this life. It seemed as improbable as the survival of one of those late-spring butterflies—you know, those little white ones—I sometimes saw wobbling through the air, always just millimeters away from smacking itself against a windshield.

When I was pregnant with my son, we were told that he might have a very serious heart condition. The doctors' dire prediction proved false. He has an insignificant valve abnormality that simply needs to be followed by regular exams. Now at seventeen, his heart and valve have grown along with him. Still when I say, "Good night, I love you, see you in the morning," I remember the gripping fear of loss. But at the age of eight, when he begged to go to sleep-away camp like his big sister, we let him go.

An explosion of new technology in baby monitors can be understood in context of these fears of loss. In one, a teddy bear with a camera in its nose hooks up to a TV, allowing parents to watch their baby's every move. One product is actually worn against the baby's skin and measures heart rate and respirations. Certainly if a baby has an identified medical condition, monitoring of heart rate and respirations may be indicated. But these monitors need to be used carefully and under supervision of a doctor. For a baby who has no such identified risk, there is no reason to monitor him. Putting a child under the age of six months to sleep on his back does more to protect him than any baby monitor.

I wonder whether these products are a kind of metaphor for a culture that does not allow space or time for accepting and processing painful feelings. When a parent seeks help for a child who is struggling, whatever the story, feelings of loss, while often not acknowledged or expressed, are front and center. Parents may mourn the imagined child, for whom life, both for them and for him, was going to be easy. Letting go of this wish for a child to be someone other than who he is enables parents to be fully present to let the child grow and develop, to see who he will become.

Pregnancy Loss, Infertility, and Unprocessed Grief

"Did you have any difficulty conceiving?" I often find that simply asking this question, before focusing on the "behavior problem" of the child whom parents have brought for evaluation, releases a flood of deep feelings related to infertility, pregnancy loss, or both.

I still vividly recall, over eighteen years later, my own family's well-meaning reassurances of "Don't worry you'll get pregnant again," that seemed so remote from the pain I felt following an early miscarriage. As a culture we often do not recognize the deep significance and impact of pregnancy loss. A recent study revealed that depression and anxiety following a miscarriage might last for almost three years, even after the birth of a healthy baby. Both parents and clinicians may expect that once a healthy baby is born, these feelings will go away. But without an opportunity to mourn this loss, to move through the pain and sorrow, these feelings of fear and sadness may persist. When they do, they may be labeled as anxiety and depression. They may get in the way of being present with a healthy baby.

One mother told me about having lost a baby at term and then suffering with severe postpartum depression when her healthy child was born a year later. In another case, a five-year-old boy I saw struggled with severe separation anxiety. At first, the focus of our work was on what to do to get him to sleep in his own room. But as we got to know each other, his mother, for the first time, spoke openly about her grief over a miscarriage when her son, an only child, was three. The little boy, it turned out, was worried about his mother. At the root of his separation anxiety was a wish to protect his mother from feeling sad. One young woman had been treated for many years for ADHD, for distracted and impulsive behavior. Only when she experienced a significant decline in her mental health did the story come to light that she had a brother who was stillborn about a year before her birth. During her early years, her mother had suffered prolonged severe depression in the face of this loss, which was never acknowledged or spoken about.

A lovely and important blog *Pregnancy After Loss Support* offers parents raising a child in the wake of loss a space to acknowledge and share these complex feelings. In one post, a mother eloquently captures the effects of this experience on a relationship with a subsequent child. She speaks to the Fed Ex man who reprimanded her for letting her son run ahead of her.

Mr. Fed Ex man, here's what you *don't* know about the scene you witnessed that morning. You don't know how difficult it is for me to let my boy go. That while he was in my womb I worried about how much longer he would stay there for nearly every minute of every day. You don't know that since he was born he has had the ability to look at me with his clear blue eyes and silently send me the message that his soul is old and wise— something that can immediately snap me back to the miracle of our relationship together. You don't know that watching him grow up and become more independent is simultaneously a pride and joy of my life as much as it is a constant grief process, watching him transform through layers of himself.

The pain and loss intimately intertwined with infertility treatment may similarly go unrecognized, especially once a healthy baby is born. However, evidence suggests that the effects may persist. A recent study in Denmark demonstrated a 33 percent increased risk of a range of psychiatric disorders in children whose mothers had been treated for infertility. The authors do not offer a cause, but postulate that the increased risk is related not to the treatments, but to the mother's reactions to the infertility itself. These "psychiatric disorders" may represent a lingering sense of loss carried into the next generation.

A mother, and also a father who, while not experiencing the physical assaults of infertility treatments, certainly shares in the emotional trauma, may come to the experience of parenthood with a range of significant vulnerabilities. Anxiety over the health of a new baby, no matter how much reassurance well-intentioned professionals offer, may be unrelenting. Repeated loss, as often occurs in the process of infertility treatment, not only with every period, but sometimes with early pregnancy loss, may lead parents, in an adaptive effort to protect themselves from further loss, to disengage emotionally. Parents may not allow themselves to surrender, to fall in love with the new baby. They also may simply be emotionally exhausted.

This finding of increased risk of psychiatric disorders in children might alarm parents who are already stressed by the process of infertility treatment. But, as was shown in the chapter on listening to babies, rather than alarm, this knowledge might offer opportunity for prevention. In an ideal world, parents who have children in the wake of infertility might receive some extra time and attention. Offering space to express feelings of grief and fear of loss, and to consider their effect on a newly formed family, might go a long way toward preventing problems in the future.

Unbearable Loss and the Replacement Child

Mental health professionals often speak about a "replacement child." These are individuals, whether adult or child, who were born following the death of a previous child. Mourning the loss of a child is never finished. It is a grief that cannot be processed. But when feelings of sadness and grief go unexpressed, they may reverberate in ways that cause trouble for other relationships.

Emily brought her son Michael to see me when he was three and a half months old. He had been born one month premature, but it was clear from a first glance that he was doing well. I remember noticing that his mother was so close, physically close. She hovered over him, but did not pick him up and seemed reluctant to let me near him.

He was a robust little boy who gave a big smile as he intently followed his mother's face. Emily, petite and soft spoken, told me she felt he was doing well. So well, in fact, that she was attributing qualities to him for which he seemed too young. "It's good for him to comfort himself, right? I should let him cry, right?" She seemed anxious.

About a year earlier, Emily had lost a baby, Christopher she called him, in her ninth month of pregnancy, when she was in a car accident. She conceived again almost immediately. And here was this miracle baby. I watched Michael sleeping in his blue jumper. Even with his full, round baby cheeks, he seemed so small and vulnerable.

"He's doing great," I said. Emily continued to wear that uncertain look as I tried to reassure her. She asked about sleep. "Is it okay if he is still in our bed? Is it good for bonding?" she asked. I was puzzled by this question and paused, asking her to tell me what she meant.

"Is he bonded to me?" she asked. I started to attempt an answer when she interrupted me. "Can you bond before birth? I mean I bonded to Christopher, but he died. I didn't let myself bond to Michael when I was carrying him."

I felt a tingling in my arms and a clutching in my chest. Tears came to my eyes as I watched them run freely down Emily's cheeks. We sat quietly for a while, living in the unbearable pain of her loss.

Emily was recognizing that getting pregnant so quickly might have prevented her from doing the difficult work of mourning the loss of her first child. She said to me, "I feel like I can't give all of myself to Michael. I have to hold back to protect myself." At that visit with me, perhaps fortified by our moment of connection, she found the courage to face this task of grieving. She recognized it was critically important not only for herself, but for her relationship with her infant son.

An op-ed in the *New York Times* captures the way in which cultural expectations may lead to blocked mourning. Ironically titled

"Getting Grief Right," the piece offers a beautiful example of the need for space and time to tell the story; to feel safe with deep sadness. The author, a psychotherapist, describes a patient who had lost a child to sudden infant death syndrome, and was surprised that after six months she was still suffering. In fact, another doctor had diagnosed her with depression and prescribed medication. The author of the piece, who speaks from experience as he, too, had lost a child, instead of asking about her symptoms, asks her to tell the story of her daughter. He writes:

> At this point in her story Mary finally began to weep, intensely so. She seemed surprised by the waves of emotion that washed over her. It was the first time since the death that the sadness had poured forth in that way. She said she had never told the story of her daughter from conception to death in one sitting . . . Her loss was now part of her story, one to claim and cherish, not a painful event to try to put in the past.

Intergenerational Transmission of Loss

When these feelings have not been given space and time to be heard, they may cause trouble in subsequent generations. Ben's story offers an example. Ben's father, John, made the first appointment. "He never listens to me," he told me on the phone, followed by, "I need your help to make him listen." Six-year-old Ben not only preferred to be with his mother, Sara, but was also frequently and openly rejecting of his father. Sara had no troubles with Ben, and at first declined to come. But as I usually do, I asked to first meet with both parents together. John was outwardly professional appearing in his elegant business suit, yet his distraught demeanor communicated despair over his relationship with his son. Sara, in contrast sat calmly beside him, seemingly nonplussed by the situation.

I learned that Ben was very close with his maternal grandmother, as was Sara. They were like a threesome that John felt unable to penetrate. Especially distressing to John was the fact that this situation did not trouble Sara in the least. She was dismissively reassuring of his worries about the increasing alienation he felt from his son. But after a couple of hour-long visits together, when both parents had grown to understand that I was curious but not judgmental, the following story emerged.

Sara's older brother, also named Ben, had died at birth, a couple of years before Sara was born. At the end of her pregnancy, she had a dream that her brother appeared and said to her, "I'm coming to be with you." It was because of this dream that she named her son Ben. Ben was a "replacement child," not of his parents, but from a previous generation. Sara had grown up in the shadow of her mother's grief over the loss of her first child. With the birth of Ben, Sara could, in a sense, rescue her mother from this grief. Ben could be the great healer, giving Sara back both her mother and her dead brother. All of this, however, was likely occurring out of awareness, or to use the Freudian term, in her unconscious.

With this story, John had new insight into his troubles with his son. His wife and mother-in-law, united in their loss, had effectively shut him out. The underlying problem was not in the relationship between John and Ben, but in this web of grief and loss.

This knowledge in itself brought great relief, as John felt the full burden of responsibility for his troubled relationship with his son lifted. Ben's behavior, his "not listening," was a form of communication. He was acting out the role his mother envisioned for him. John had misinterpreted his behavior as a rejection, and responded with anger, setting in place a pattern of miscommunication. Now that he could reinterpret the meaning of this behavior, he could react less with anger and more with calm limit setting, to which Ben quickly responded with significant improvement in his behavior. Sara, now aware of how her son had, in a sense, stood in for her dead brother, was able to support the healing relationship between her husband and son.

Until Sara and John had an opportunity to tell this story, Sara could not see Ben as himself. If a child represents someone else, he may develop what Winnicott called a "false self" out of a desire to comply with his parents' needs. Ben, in a way that was also unconscious, was becoming what his mother and grandmother needed him to be. He complied with his mother and grandmother's need to replace their lost brother and son, and the intense intimacy this demanded made him complicit with excluding his father.

Now that the story had been brought to light, John's relationship with his son could be repaired. Had it not been told, the distance between Ben and his father might have increased, unchecked, having unknown long-term effects on all of the relationships in the family. Ben might have grown up without a meaningful relationship with his father. One could imagine that as an adult, symptoms of this disturbed relationship might have surfaced, perhaps when he himself had a son. When a source of the loss is unacknowledged, symptoms may persist for generations. The original story becomes further distorted and hard to recognize.

A Second Chance

Many of the patients who come to the Austen Riggs Center have been receiving psychiatric care unsuccessfully for years. They have carried multiple psychiatric diagnoses and been treated with multiple psychiatric medications. The unique open setting of this hospital makes ample time and space to tell the family stories that may never have been told or heard. There is an opportunity to connect symptoms with long-buried and unmourned losses.

A Riggs publication, *A Patient's Perspective*, offers a composite (disguised to protect confidentiality) yet representative story of a patient, a young woman with a history of substance abuse and multiple psychiatric diagnoses prior to coming to Riggs. Of a family treatment session this patient writes:

> I learned a lot about my family that I did not know. My grandmother had been abandoned as a child and brought up by an aunt, my father had a difficult relationship with his own father and my parents had all this unresolved anger and grief and guilt about having to take care of my grandmother toward the end of her life and never really mourned her death. I really had no idea how hard things had been for my grandmother or my parents and hearing about their struggles gave me a different perspective. I learned I was the one who had collapsed under the weight of the losses in my family and as long as I was the "patient" in my family, no one else had to confront their own losses and grief.

This kind of story is not only typical of the patients who have the opportunity to receive treatment at Riggs, but likely also true of many with mental illness who do not.

French psychoanalysts Françoise Davoine and Jean-Max Gaudillière's book, *History Beyond Trauma* is subtitled, "Whereof one cannot speak, thereof one cannot stay silent." They argue that personal stories of trauma, if not told in words, emerge as mental illness. They make the distinction between "big history," as in the context of societal conflict and war, and individual family history, noting that the second can sometimes be a reverberation of the first.

Singer-songwriter Dar Williams expresses this phenomenon beautifully in her song "After All." With powerful feelings conveyed through the music itself, she describes how she came to understand her depression as a reverberation of her own parents' history, both their individual family story and their "big history." In her introduction to a live recording, she expresses surprise to have discovered a large community of people who could relate to her experience.

> *Well the whole truth*
> *It's like the story of a wave unfurled*

To heal herself, she needed to learn that story.
> *And if I was to sleep*
> *I knew my family had more truth to tell*
> *So I traveled down a whispering well*
> *To know myself through them*

She recognizes the importance of moving through grief.
> *I know they tried to keep their pain from me*
> *They could not see what it was for*

The lyrics indicate that Williams has come to understand some of the "big history."
> *But now I'm sleeping fine*
> *Sometimes the truth is like a second chance*
> *I am the daughter of a great romance*
> *And they are the children of the war.*

Once she has "traveled down that whispering well," she is able to find peace; to join the world of the living. The label of depression, in the absence of time and space to tell the story, might have served to silence the pain, of both Williams and her parents. In contrast, by learning the story she moved through the pain and came to a new closeness and connection.

The Value of Family Stories

A child comes in to the world with his full screaming self, demanding to be recognized. But parents may be held back from full recognition by painful family history. As we have seen, "behavior problems" may be a child's efforts to communicate, "I need you to deal with this so you will be free to be with me."

Yet resistance to telling family stories can be high. Parents may feel that exploring their own history to understand their child's behavior means that any current problems are their "fault." Guilt, the wish to avoid painful memories, as well as fear that the feelings will not be understood, all contribute to what may be intense ambivalence about exploring the past.

Making time to hear the parent's story is thus an essential part of helping a child. In one paper, "Speaking Silence," psychologist Robyn Fivush of Emory University quotes philosopher Susan Brison, "In order to construct self-narratives we need not only the words with which to tell our stories, but also an audience able and willing to hear us and to understand our words as we intend them."

Research by Fivush and Marshall Duke, also at Emory, described in a *New York Times* article, "The Family Stories That Bind Us," offers evidence that a child's knowledge of family history, of his family's story, is associated with resilience, positive self-esteem, and overall mental health. The correlation is particularly high when the narrative includes both successes and hardship—what they refer to as an "oscillating narrative." This knowledge of his family's story gives a child what researchers have termed an "intergenerational self."

While this research shows a correlation between a child's knowledge of family history and positive self-esteem, it does not explain just how that knowledge contributes to healthy development. I wonder whether the causal link is related to the parents' own mourning process and subsequent ability to move their own issues off their child, thus recognizing and supporting what Winnicott would call his true self. When parents can acknowledge their losses and failures, as well as achievements, they are free to see the child as himself. In contrast, when troublesome feelings are held in, particularly when there is a kind of blocked mourning for a long-buried loss, the child may go unseen. His desire to connect may find expression through his behavior.

Listening with Hope

When I was nine years old, I was painfully shy and inhibited. Had I been a child today, I might have been diagnosed with social anxiety disorder, and perhaps placed on an SSRI (selective serotonin reuptake inhibitor). But instead, under the influence of parents who subscribed to Socrates's belief that "the unexamined life is not worth living," I set upon a journey to discover the cause of these symptoms.

I now know that nine was the age of my father when Hitler came to power. I grew up in the shadow of a story my father had not told. His losses in the Holocaust, of family, friends, and country, lived in me. The silence of this untold story was a gap between us. His loss became my loss.

It took two generations for this story to begin to be told, and the courage of my son in asking his grandfather to break the silence. In

March 2012, my then eighty-eight-year-old father spoke with Eli's eighth grade class following its visit to the Holocaust Museum in Washington, DC.

He sat on a folding chair on the bare school auditorium stage, before an audience of transfixed young teenagers. He spoke for a full hour, without pausing for even a drink of water. He described growing up in Germany under the rise of Hitler and his escape as a teenager through a program bringing unaccompanied children to the United States, where he became a citizen. He told the story of his miraculous rescue of his parents from a concentration camp at the end of the war when, having returned to Germany as a soldier with the US Army, he happened to be stationed near his hometown. After not knowing what had happened to his parents for close to five years, he was able to discover their whereabouts from the town's former mayor. His commanding officer gave him permission to fly a small plane to Theresienstadt, where he found them and was then able to bring them to safety.

Both my mother and father, in a highly adaptive way, display a kind of relentless optimism, an insistence that everything is "great." In a well-meaning effort to protect him, my mother clearly communicated her conviction that speaking at Eli's school could cause my father harm. But having found my own voice (as an only child the decision was mine alone), I overcame my fears that something terrible would happen to him that day, and the plan went forward.

Afterward, he was positively exhilarated. The event opened up a part of him I had never seen. This brief encounter with the depth of his experience allowed a new connection to begin to form between us. Hungry for more, I suggested we write a book together. But this effort, while initially met by great enthusiasm, soon brought me back to that familiar place of silence. When I tried to talk with him, I heard a few more stories, but the cracking in his voice revealed a glimpse of the unbearable pain behind his experience, and soon he could say no more.

So, I set out to tell his story through mine. At first the book was going to be about mourning. Recognizing how often loss is at the root of "behavior problems" in children, my aim was to show the significance of mourning in healing.

Yet my editor balked at this idea. Was there a "right" way to mourn? Such a book might feel too prescriptive. But what was it, she asked, that allowed these transformative moments to happen in my office where parents shed tears, and in doing so discovered meaningful connection with their children? I mentioned a blog post I had written, entitled "Space and Time Is the Treatment." "That's it!" she cried, practically jumping out of her chair. A book about space and time for listening was born.

Had I been medicated for social anxiety at the age of nine, there is a good chance that neither my father's nor many of the stories in this book would have been heard. Telling my story took a lot of time. The therapist I finally connected with at the age of forty gave me a safe space to shed rivers of tears, in a sense mourning for my father, both his loss and mine. Now by helping other parents to mourn loss and so connect with their young children, the silence around my father's story has found expression in my clinical work, and in this book.

Ten

Listening with Courage: The Value of Uncertainty

Creativity requires the courage to let go of certainty.

—*Erich Fromm*

With an openness to let a story unfold, it never ceases to amaze me what we can discover when we approach a "problem behavior" from a stance of inquiry, of not knowing. Kyra came to see me for sleep problems. After fifteen months of waking every two to three hours to nurse her son Henry, she was crumbling in the face of severe sleep deprivation. At first contained and controlled, with a logical determination to solve the problem, she asked for advice about what to do. She knew there was no way to teach him to sleep through the night unless she stopped the nighttime nursing, but, she told me, she was unable to wean Henry for fear of causing him harm. Instead of giving reassurance or advice, I noticed this quandary she was in, and asked her to explain how she thought she might "cause him harm." As I often find, this stance of curiosity led to a dramatic shift in her posture, tone, and thinking. As she first contemplated, and then began to explain, what lay behind this fear, her true feelings emerged. Her face and body softened; she wept through her words as she told the story of the sudden death of her younger brother, for whom her son was named. Though intellectually she knew her brother's death in a boating accident was not her fault, she had been left with a gripping doubt. She would have to come to terms with these feelings, but she already saw that the worry about "causing harm" was not about Henry. We were both moved, not only by the discovery of this untold story hidden behind the symptom, but also by how powerfully transformative this moment felt.

Once the feelings were put in their rightful place, Kyra was able to wean Henry off his nighttime nursing. He began to sleep through the night, and a previously elusive feeling of peace descended over the entire family.

"I know how you feel," a common well-intentioned, yet sometimes jarring expression of sympathy, stands in contrast to empathy, a kind of not-knowing. In her highly acclaimed collection of essays, *The Empathy Exams*, Leslie Jamison captures this idea well, writing: "Empathy requires inquiry as much as imagination. Empathy requires knowing you know nothing. Empathy means acknowledging a horizon of context that extends perpetually beyond what you can see . . ." When we aim to imagine our way in to another person's experience while acknowledging we can't really know, we can join them, be present with them in a way that is central to growth and healing.

Winnicott identified the role of uncertainty in the development of the true self, from the earliest months of life. Following the stage of total preoccupation, when the mother anticipates the helpless infant's every need, comes an essential time when she can't and should not do so. As the child gains increased competence and begins to develop into her own separate person, the mother will naturally be unsure of what she needs. The good-enough mother is not perfect, and these very imperfections give the child space to grow into herself. Winnicott writes:

> As soon as the mother and infant are separate, from the infant's point of view, then it will be noted that the mother tends to change her attitude. It is as if she now realizes that the infant no longer expects the condition in which there is an almost magical understanding of need. It could be said that if she now knows too well what the infant needs, this is magic, and forms no basis for [a] relationship.

Through these earliest mismatches, these "failures," or moments of not-knowing, a child is learning to tolerate the inevitable uncertainties inherent in human relationships. In a paper entitled "On Curiosity," psychoanalyst Ed Shapiro captures the role of uncertainty in development of the true self. He writes of the mother:

> She must be able to suspend her conviction about the accuracy of her empathy (i.e. suspend her certainty) in order to provide *an open space in her mind* into which her child's more differentiated image can develop. In this undefined and potential space the child is given the freedom to define himself in his own way, with his own capabilities.

The Need for Patience

When a child struggles, parents may be under great pressure to name the problem. But it takes time for a story to unfold. An approach that requires patience flies in the face of the current health-care system where payments are contingent on labels. The need to have a diagnosis so as to get "services" may lead us prematurely to name something as an illness before a child has a chance, together with her parents, to work out her own way of handling the struggle.

Uncertainty is inherent in the search to finding meaning in behavior. For a rapidly developing child, the time is relatively short, but for a parent this uncertainty can be difficult to bear, particularly in our quick-fix society. For example, the kind of free-form, playful visit I describe in Chapter 5 may initially cause parents significant anxiety, as they expect a more formal assessment. They may implore their child, "Talk to the doctor, Joey!" But if we just stick with a slow pace—"not knowing what's going on," as the trainee observing Winnicott described—the visit often reveals significant insight and meaning.

Rather than offer time and space for the nuances, complexities, and uncertainties of human behavior and relationships, the DSM, with its diagnoses of disorders based on symptoms, often leading to prescribing of medication, creates an aura of certainty, as in "You have X and the treatment is Y." Early childhood is a time of massive developmental shifts. When we name a problem in a young child as a "disorder," we run the risk of acting before the full picture has come into focus. Parents, clinicians, and teachers may see a child's behavior as part of an illness, rather than part of an emerging self.

When a young child is given a diagnostic label, in Winnicott's words she may come to "comply" with this adult definition of her experience and live up to her diagnosis. Winnicott's view includes a belief that "living creatively is a healthy state, and that compliance is a sick basis for life."

In 1959, in the wake of the first iteration of the diagnostic and statistical manual, DSM I, Winnicott was already worried about the way these diagnostic labels were being used. He saw how a psychiatrist, looking at an individual at a specific moment in time, such as when a crisis or a hospitalization occurs, might fail to recognize the individual's history and context. While Winnicott recognized the value of classification, he also saw the need to incorporate what he calls the "environment," or the relationships that form the context of a person's development. He saw how the label given to an individual patient would change as the story unfolded.

The psychiatric diagnoses we see rising exponentially today have unintended consequences for children in a system of care that does not have time and space to listen to the story. When Winnicott was writing, the vast array of psychiatric medications to treat these "illnesses" did not yet exist. Nor did he practice in the confines of a complex health insurance industry that created the fifteen-minute medication check. The urgency of his message is now magnified in the setting of these societal shifts. Focus on swift diagnosis and prescribing of medication may promote a kind of compliance that can suppress a child's healthy development.

Brain Science and the Search for Certainty

Just like the digital codes of replicating life held within DNA, the brain's fundamental secret will be laid open one day. But even when it has, the wonder will remain, that mere wet stuff can make this bright inward cinema of thought, of sight and sound and touch bound into a vivid illusion of instantaneous present, with a self, another brightly wrought illusion, hovering like a ghost at its centre. Could it ever be explained, how matter becomes conscious?

In these words, Ian McEwan, in his novel *Saturday*, about a day in the life of a neurosurgeon, expresses awe at the human mind. The beauty of his words, in turn, inspires awe for his mind's creative capacity. Psychologist Gary Marcus in a *New York Times* op-ed, calls attention to "the trouble with brain science." Perhaps inspired by this very piece of writing, he refers to the lack of a bridge between neuroscience and psychology comparable to the bridge between genetics and living beings that discovery of the double helix provided.

But, in fact, we do have one bridge, as exemplified by the act of reading this vivid description. Reading that passage puts us in relationship with its author. The bridge is human connection. We will never understand the brain just by looking at the brain. The brain only makes sense in the context of communication. When seen in this light, listening could be the bridge between neuroscience and psychology.

Former NIMH (National Institute of Mental Health) director Thomas Insel recently called for a study of the neuroscience of mental illness in the same way we study cancer, food allergies, and diabetes. Shortly before the *DSM 5* was published, he dealt what seemed to be a deathblow, declaring that they would no longer fund research based on the *DSM* system of diagnosis. He expressed a goal to reshape the direction of psychiatric research to focus on biology, genetics, and neuroscience so that scientists can define disorders by their causes, rather than their symptoms. The NIMH is in the process of developing an elegant and complex system called the RDoC, or Research Domain Criteria, that aims to classify mental disorders objectively by observable behaviors and neurobiological measures. This system may represent an improvement over the *DSM* system as it does acknowledge developmental and environmental effects. But the overall emphasis is on the study of neural circuits. In an article about psychiatric medication use in children, in which he compared childhood emotional and behavioral problems to diabetes and food allergies, Insel referred to biomarkers. He seemed to be looking to the day when we may be able to test for mental illness in children with a blood test or a brain scan.

The wish to equate psychological experience with physical illness, as exemplified by an oft-used phrase, "Depression is like diabetes," ostensibly comes from a wish to destigmatize emotional suffering (as well as obtain parity, or equal insurance coverage). This comparison is an effort to apply certainty to situations ripe with uncertainty. But, in fact, it may have the opposite effect, as it devalues the role of human relationships and the complexity of the human mind. Recent research reveals that biological explanations of mental illness do not decrease, and may increase, public perceptions of stigma. In addition, clinician empathy has been found to decrease in the face of such explanations. A 2014 study from the department of psychology at Yale University states that "biological accounts of psychopathology can exacerbate perceptions of patients as abnormal, distinct from the rest of the population, meriting social exclusion, and even less than fully human."

Diabetes is a disorder of insulin metabolism. Insulin is produced in the pancreas. Unlike the brain, the pancreas has no corresponding mind with thoughts and feelings. The pancreas does not love. It does not grieve, nor does it produce great literature. In his tome on depression, *The Noonday Demon*, Andrew Solomon articulates this idea beautifully. He writes:

> Although depression is described by the popular press and the pharmaceutical industry as though it were a single effect illness such as diabetes, it is not. Indeed, it is strikingly dissimilar to

diabetes. Diabetics produce insufficient insulin, and diabetes is treated by increasing and stabilizing insulin in the bloodstream. Depression is *not* the consequence of a reduced level of anything we can now measure . . . "I'm depressed but it's just chemical" is a sentence equivalent to "I'm murderous but it's just chemical" or "I'm intelligent but it's just chemical." Everything about a person is just chemical if one wants to think in those terms . . . The sun shines brightly and that's just chemical too, and it's chemical that rocks are hard, and that the sea is salt, and that certain springtime afternoons carry in their gentle breezes a quality of nostalgia that stir the heart to longings and imaginings kept dormant by the snows of a long winter.

Locating the problem in the brain offers a sense of certainty. In contrast, recognizing the complex connections among brain, mind, behavior, and feelings calls for tolerance of uncertainty. Friends, family, and professionals can help parents to manage uncertainty and to contain the inevitable anxiety that accompanies a period of not-knowing. However, in the absence of that kind of support, or what Winnicott termed a "holding environment," that allows a child's development to unfold, certainty may feel preferable.

Preschool Depression: A Need for Caution

Research by Dr. Joan Luby at Washington University exemplifies the disease model of biological psychiatry. The danger of this model is the certainty with which young children are labeled with major psychiatric disorders. Luby and her research team have evidence of brain differences in children with behavior that falls under the category of Major Depressive Disorder as defined by the DSM. A recent study showed that at age six, children who had received a diagnosis of preschool depression had smaller volumes of a structure called the insula than do children who did not have this diagnosis. Furthermore, children who exhibit what they call "pathological guilt" were more likely to have a smaller volume of the insula. Their conclusions are twofold. One is that the insula is implicated as a biomarker for major depression. The second is that helping children to "manage" symptoms of "pathological guilt" might offer a path to prevention.

This interpretation sounds alarm bells for me. While Luby's group does not advocate for pharmacological treatment of depression, vulnerability to marketing efforts by the pharmaceutical industry is inherent in labeling a young child with this major psychiatric disorder. I hope to sound these bells before the *DSM* defined preschool depression goes the way of ADHD, with children being medicated in the absence of space and time to listen to the story, to understand behavior not as a symptom of a "disorder," but as a form of communication.

While Luby and her group call attention to the need to support children who are struggling in the preschool years, and advocate for interventions that support parent-child relationships as a form of prevention, the danger of this model lies in its direct path from symptoms to a *DSM*-diagnosed disorder. Her research offers a classic example of being stuck in a medical model of disease. In a recent study, Luby and her team identify how preschoolers with what they call "high-intensity defiant behavior" and "high-intensity tantrums" are more likely to be diagnosed with conduct disorder. However, as we have seen, tantrums are a form of communication. The so-called conduct disorder may result when that communication is not heard. Lack of an understanding response, rather than the tantrums themselves, may be the link to later mental health problems.

Four-year-old Isabel's parents, Paul and Andrea, were distraught that she often described herself as "bad," even on occasion saying, "I hate myself." She quickly accepted blame when something went wrong. When I opened the first visit, at which Isabel was not present, with, "Start wherever you'd like," Isabel's mother took the lead while Paul sat quietly, his body language communicating a kind of awkwardness and disconnection, as if he felt he didn't really belong. Yet when I took advantage of a pause in Andrea's story to address him directly with a question, he relaxed and opened up. He seemed relieved to have the opportunity to share his feelings and experience. He told me the following story. When Paul misbehaved as a child, his father would slap him across the face, berating him for being, "an embarrassment to the family." He shared vivid memories, accompanied by deep feelings of shame and humiliation, of being grabbed by the ear and dragged away from family gatherings. Now a father himself, with no other model for discipline, he found himself repeating the same pattern with his own daughter. "What's wrong with you?" he would shout. Her frequent meltdowns, the reason for the visit with me, precipitated not only yelling and commands of "Go to your room" but also such statements as "Why can't you be more like your baby brother?" At first he surprised himself by talking so openly about his past. Rarely, he told me, did he have a chance to talk about his feelings in this way. He recognized that our conversation gave him a new way to understand his ongoing conflicts with his daughter.

Isabel, temperamentally more like her mother than her father, was very sensitive and easily disorganized, a quality she displayed since birth, in contrast to her "easy" baby brother. Both parents acknowledged deep conflict over discipline. Andrea grew up in a home that, unlike Paul's, had little discipline. "But," she said, "I was a 'good girl,' so it wasn't a problem." Now Paul frequently blamed Isabel's behavior on Andrea's lax discipline, leading to an atmosphere of tension in the home, aggravated by the chronic sleep deprivation accompanying the arrival of a new baby.

I wonder whether what Luby and colleagues are calling "pathological guilt" is actually shame. Guilt can be a normal and healthy emotional experience. "I'm guilty" can also mean "I'm responsible." Shame, in contrast, is always pathological and can have destructive effects on emotional development. But without an opportunity to hear the family story, it is impossible to distinguish between the two. Knowing Paul's story, we can understand it as a kind of intergenerational transmission of shame. Isabel's sad feelings and expressions of low self-esteem were a communication of distress at an environment of rage, directed both at her and between her parents. One can understand her feelings and behavior not as an illness but as an adaptive effort to change the situation.

This experience of shame might very well have an impact on the growth of the insula. Luby's conclusions imply that a person has a small insula in the same way one might have an abnormal pancreas. But as we have seen, the brain grows in relationships. When we do not know the full story, we should not draw conclusions from brain scans. Perhaps if this pattern were to continue in Isabel's family, a brain scan in a few years might show that Isabel has a smaller insula than her brother, though even that finding might represent a combination of genetic and experiential factors. Research in biological psychiatry that connects "symptoms" and "disorders" with brain scans, without fully exploring the context of relationships, fails to form the bridge between psychology and neuroscience.

Prevention does not lie in teaching Isabel, as Luby's team recommends, to "manage her guilt." This approach represents a devaluing of the healing power of human connection, a direct result of the *DSM* illness model that places the problem squarely in the child. Support of parent-child relationships must include opportunity for listening and discovering meaning.

Once Paul had an opportunity to identify the source of his behavior in his own history, he felt heard and understood, and so was better able to listen to his daughter. He saw not only the flaws in the discipline he had received and inadvertently copied, but also how his approach was particularly difficult for Isabel, given her sensitive nature. Andrea and Paul appreciated how their own conflict, even when they tried to keep it from their children, raised the level of tension in the home. In the normal frenzy of activity that occurs in a household with a new baby, they had no time or space to reflect on these problems.

In his paper "On Curiosity," Shapiro uses the term "pathological certainty" to refer to the way, in cases of severe psychopathology, "family members are often extraordinarily certain that they know, understand, and can speak for the experience of other family members without further discussion or question." Giving young children a diagnosis of major depression based on "symptoms" and drawing conclusions based on brain scans can be understood as an institutionalized form of pathological certainty. In contrast, by listening with curiosity and letting the story unfold, we have opportunity to understand the meaning of behavior in all its complexity. There are as many variations to the stories behind "symptoms of depression," as there are families.

Many professionals who advocate for diagnosing depression in the preschool age group argue that the alternative is to minimize the problem, and to deny that young children do suffer with deep feelings of sadness. But listening, rather than labeling, is the opposite of denial. When we listen to young children and their parents, we validate and respect the full range of their powerful emotions.

Diagnostic Certainty and ADHD

Recently I spoke with Cora, mother of eleven-year-old Skylar, whose teachers were wondering about ADHD and suggesting medication. Cora reflected on her daughter's multiple talents; she had a beautiful voice and could express herself calmly and clearly through music. While team sports were difficult, she excelled at ice skating, skiing, and running, all activities that brought out the best in her. She was struggling with the increasingly complex social dynamics of middle school. Cora wanted to think carefully about this next step in supporting her daughter's development. Yet when she called Skylar's pediatrician to schedule a time to discuss these issues, she was told by the receptionist that before she could even make an appointment, which the receptionist termed an "ADHD evaluation," she needed to fill out, and have the teacher fill out, the ADHD rating scales. The question being asked was not "How do we understand the challenges Skylar is experiencing," but rather "Does she or does she not have ADHD?" The label came before the opportunity to think about and find meaning in Skylar's behavior. Cora spoke thoughtfully about older family members with similar traits who had adapted to their quirks and become scientists and writers. Cora longed to give her daughter an opportunity to recognize and overcome her struggles in a healthy and adaptive way. But she felt cornered into naming the problem before they even began to explore its source.

Many clinicians, in explaining medication to parents and children, make an analogy between ADHD and nearsightedness, with medication analogous to glasses. This analogy underscores the fallacy of certainty with regard to psychiatric diagnosis in children. We have very specific knowledge of the biology of nearsightedness, and the mechanism by which glasses correct abnormal vision. An ophthalmologist can measure the length of the eye and know, based on specific results, the exact prescription needed. She can take measurements over time adjusting the prescription in exact parallel with anatomic changes.

There is no corresponding known specific biology, or biomarker, known for what we call ADHD. There is evidence of a genetic basis to the ability to regulate attention. However, there is no gene for ADHD. In fact, National Institutes of Health–funded researchers have recently discovered that people with disorders traditionally thought to be distinct—autism, ADHD, bipolar disorder, major depression, and schizophrenia—have similar genetic variations on the same chromosomes.

While we have some knowledge of neurochemistry and structures of the brain responsible for regulation of attention, behavior, and emotion, there is no specific brain abnormality that corresponds to this entity we call ADHD. The measurement of symptoms, and corresponding adjustment of medications, guided by subjective descriptions of behavior, is far from exact.

A colleague of mine has proposed an approach he terms "deconstructing" ADHD. Jane's story offers an example.

"I just need to know if she has ADHD," Dara asked anxiously of their three-year-old daughter Jane at our first visit, while her wife Lori held their infant son Ben on her lap. Dara, Jane's biological mother, had herself been recently diagnosed. I learned that Dara had struggled terribly as a young child, her flighty nature leading her strict parents to direct constant anger and disapproval at her. When pregnant, Dara felt the high activity level of her unborn child and worried that she, too, might have this disorder. She not only closely identified with her young daughter, but also felt terrible guilt that the challenges they were experiencing might be her "fault." As I opened up the conversation, she kept insisting that I tell her with certainty whether Jane did or did not have ADHD. If the answer was yes, then they could "do something now." If the answer was no, they presumably could feel relief and move on.

But as we got toward the end of the visit, Lori began to express some uncertainty about this "either-or" view. When I encouraged her to explain, she spoke of Jane's intense curiosity and ability to notice things. Dara had the same traits, Lori told me, which she put to good use in her successful career as an architect. But Jane got easily overwhelmed when there was a lot of stimulation, as there had been recently with the arrival of the new baby. Not only would she spiral into high activity, but also climb into potentially dangerous spots, with her behavior quickly escalating into an explosive meltdown. Lori turned to her wife and gently asked Dara whether she noticed this pattern. Dara said yes, acknowledging that her anxiety got the better of her in these situations and she was quick to react with anger. Lori wondered whether the increased negative attention, and lack of one-on-one time with either parent, might have exacerbated the problem. Dara agreed.

Over a number of visits we continued to deconstruct the question of ADHD, examining the different factors contributing to Jane's behavior. When I saw the whole family together, we got to experience this deconstruction in real time, leading both parents to a place of insight and direction. Ben, who had just learned to walk, was the first one in the office. He went straight to the toy shelf and began knocking things down. Next, Jane ran in to join him. The visit already felt on the verge of being out of control. Dara and Lori sat on the couch, attempting to tell me what had happened since we last met. But the situation quickly escalated. When Jane grabbed a toy from Ben and he screamed loudly in protest, Dara reprimanded her. Within seconds Jane was running around the room, then climbing on the table. When Dara went to pick her up, she kicked her mother. "This is what we're talking about," Lori explained over Ben's crying. "I'll take Jane and then you can talk with Dara." Dara agreed, relieved to be rescued from this highly stressful scene. But having a sense that this "problem" was somehow linked to Dara's relationship with her daughter, I suggested that the totally out-of-control Jane stay in the room, and Lori take Ben for a walk. It was a gamble, but it immediately paid off. For just as quickly as she had escalated into a wild child, Jane transformed back into a delightful engaged little girl. For a few minutes the three of us sat on the floor and played together, but for the rest of the visit Jane played quietly with the dollhouse while I spoke with her mother.

In that moment Dara experienced in a dramatically vivid way that Jane responded to stress—in this case of both sensory overload and need to compete with her brother for attention—with escalation in activity. Equally importantly, Dara appreciated how giving her daughter calm attention could help her calm down. Now Dara was open to hearing what Lori had been telling her about the positive qualities, including her sensitivities, she shared with her daughter, and how these qualities only became a problem in particular situations, such as the stress of both a screaming brother and angry mother. Dara could clearly see how her daughter's behavior provoked her to react in ways that were not helpful.

In our meetings, we had identified traits of high activity and distractibility in two generations, indicating a possible genetic component, a stressed relationship between mother and child that echoed conflicts in the previous generation, and sensory processing challenges in the context of a busy household with a very active and often loud baby.

Both parents began to work together to help channel Jane's intense and inquisitive nature in positive ways, and to support each other in providing the attention that both children needed. When I spoke with them a few months later, Jane was thriving in a new preschool. She was working with an occupational therapist to address her sensory sensitivities. There was no more mention of ADHD.

Many clinicians speak of what they call "straightforward ADHD," insisting that the children for whom they prescribe medication have isolated difficulty with sequencing actions and solving problems, or what is termed executive function. But if we do not take time to hear the full background, how can we possibly know? As we have seen, these often complex and multilayered stories do not emerge in the rating scales and structured diagnostic interviews based on *DSM* criteria. Once a child has been diagnosed, time for listening to the unfolding story as she grows and develops may further evaporate. In a study of over 300,000 children receiving medication for ADHD fewer than 25 percent received any kind of talk therapy; and in two hundred US counties, fewer than 1 in 10 children received any form of therapy other than medication. Another study reviewed over 1,500 charts of 188 pediatricians in different communities, finding that the vast majority—93.4 percent—of those diagnosed with ADHD were receiving medication, and only 13 percent were receiving any form of psychosocial treatment.

Eight-year-old Lexi offers an example of this typical pattern of treatment. Her parents came to see me for a consultation after two years of Lexi's being prescribed medication for ADHD, when they became concerned about its long-term effect.

Lexi had begun showing signs of distractibility and hyperactivity as soon as she entered kindergarten; her teachers couldn't manage her, and she became a regular at the principal's office. They consulted their pediatrician who did some rating scales and diagnosed ADHD. After a few months of implementing "behavior management strategies," they tried a low dose of stimulant medication and saw immediate positive change. Lexi took this formulation, with an increase in the dose midway through the year, through first grade. When she started second grade, they started the medication again. By winter, she needed a higher dose. They also were starting to see breakthrough hyperactivity and inattentiveness between the morning and afternoon doses, so the pediatrician recommended an extended release preparation. She spent that year going from medication to medication, with as they described, periods of improvement in behavior followed by escalation of what her parents, teachers, and physicians called "symptoms" of her ADHD. When I spoke on the phone with Lexi's mother to set up an appointment, she told me that she and Lexi's father had recently gotten divorced but that the pediatrician and teachers did not think it was related, as signs of ADHD had begun before the divorce.

My first thought in conversation with Lexi's parents was to wonder not only about the impact of marital conflict on her behavior, but also the impact of her behavior on the marriage. A child's inattentive, distracted, and hyperactive behavior can inevitably grate on not only the relationship between parent and child, but also relationships between parents and among siblings. As we saw in Jane's story, what may have started as a "trait" can be transformed into a "problem" in a stressful environment. Research has demonstrated that an individual might have a genetic predisposition for the behaviors associated with ADHD, but only develop what qualifies as a DSM-defined disorder in a home filled with conflict.

Furthermore, I learned in that initial conversation that despite her having been diagnosed and treated with medication for two years, there had been no exploration of the possible role of sensory processing in Lexi's current difficulties, either at home or in school.

While there is certainty when a change in glasses prescription corresponds to a change in vision, increasing a dose of medication to eliminate "difficult behavior" conveys a false certainty that the behavior is caused by the ADHD. In addition, the act of giving a prescription for psychiatric medication to a developing child may have impact, beyond the drug itself, which may go unrecognized. What does it mean to a child to take a pill to "manage" her behavior? Often discussions occur in front of a child about changing dose and formulation based on her "problem behavior." This experience, unlike changing glasses prescriptions, will inevitably have impact on that child's emerging sense of self.

Autism: A Search for "the Truth"

Several years ago, when the change in diagnostic criteria for Autism Spectrum Disorder proposed for *DSM 5* was in the news, and parents were worried that their children would lose their label and with it the help they were receiving, I wrote a blog post about the problem of giving children a diagnostic label so as to get services covered by insurance. An irate reader, Landon Bryce, a well-known speaker and advocate for people with autism, wrote a blog post in response in which he said, "Dr. Gold simply does not understand that autism is not a psychiatric disorder."

In the wake of the recent CDC (Centers for Disease Control) statistics indicating that 1 in 68 children has autism, I have been thinking a great deal about the dilemma he raised. For Bryce and I were really on exactly the same page. Both of us were calling for a respect for and valuing of difference.

Andrew Solomon beautifully articulates this perspective in his book *Far from the Tree*, when he identifies the power of unconditional love and complete acceptance of individual differences. In the chapter on autism, Solomon suggests that by hoping a child does not have autism, a parent is saying that she wishes this child did not exist and that she had a different child. However, in my clinical work, I see the exact opposite. The parents who seek evaluation for a young child who is struggling love their child unconditionally. They are motivated to understand her experience. Rather than rushing to name the problem, they long to give their child space and time to adapt to her unique abilities and challenges, to make them part of her emerging sense of self in a positive way.

While evidence points to genetic and neurobiological mechanisms in the behaviors collectively referred to as autism, it is not a known biological entity as are, using Tom Insel's examples, food allergies and diabetes. In fact part of the problem with this label, and why these discussions are inevitably highly fraught, is that a vast array of difference is subsumed under that one word. For just as there are adults like Bryce who can advocate for their uniqueness, there are severely disabled individuals, who carry the exact same diagnosis, who are unable to communicate at all. While I fundamentally agree with the perspective of Bryce and Solomon, my mind stumbles on this fact. We see this very problem in Steve Silberman's recent in-depth exploration of the question of autism as "difference" vs. "disorder" in *NeuroTribes*. In her review of the book, Jennifer Senior writes: "Many of the autistic individuals he profiles also tilt toward the exquisitely articulate, because they've helped lead a movement. . . . The consequence is that we don't see autism in some of its more devastating forms."

Winnicott's musings on the subject of autism, though written in 1966, have relevance today.

> From my point of view the invention of the term autism was a mixed blessing . . . I would like to say that once this term has been invented and applied, the stage was set for something which is slightly false, i.e. the discovery of a disease . . . Pediatricians and physically minded doctors as a whole like to think in terms of diseases which gives a tidy look to the textbooks . . . The unfortunate thing is that in matters psychological things are not like that.

Winnicott implores the reader to instead understand the child in a context of development, and of relationships, which he calls "the environmental provision." He looks beyond the symptoms of a possible disorder to the full story of a child's development, and whether this has been encouraged or hindered by early relationships and experiences.

An approach like Winnicott's may be fraught in the context of the history of "refrigerator mothers," a theory attributing autism to lack of parental warmth that has been widely discounted. Any attempt to consider the child's relational and developmental context may revive that judgmental view and be interpreted as "blaming the parent." Winnicott calls for us not to "blame," but rather to take time to look at the child's struggles in the whole context of "human emotional development." The very act of listening to the story becomes the cornerstone of treatment.

The following case offers an example of the contrast between certainty and uncertainty, and how the latter can allow for growth and healing. Lisa and Joe raised concerns with their pediatrician about their three-year-old son Pete's difficulty interacting with the other kids in preschool. He was showing increasingly inflexible behavior, with a need for strict routines. Explosive meltdowns could occur when things did not go as he expected. His teachers had raised the question of autism.

Their pediatrician, who had known Pete since he was born, had dismissed their concerns as "nothing to worry about." But, seeing that Pete's parents were nonetheless worried, he had given them my name, as well as that of a major medical center. Mine was the first available appointment, so Pete's parents got on the waiting list for an "autism evaluation" and, while they waited, began work with me.

When Pete came to visits with me, he used his remarkable verbal skills to take control. With an exuberant personality to match his head of thick brown curls, he dictated who played with whom, and who could talk when. His fun and lively play could easily fill the time, and when our conversation drifted to a difficult moment at home, such as a meltdown at a family gathering, he commanded that I stop asking questions. Not surprisingly, when parents discuss their children's "problem" behavior in front of them, it can create anxiety. Pete's way of dealing with his anxiety was to try to take charge. His rigidity and what his parents referred to as "obsessive" need for order could be seen as his brain's way of managing anxiety.

In our time together, we grew to understand that he had difficulty regulating himself in a highly stimulating environment, a quality that he had had since birth, and that he in fact shared with a number of family members. The gentle pace of our visits helped Pete and his parents make sense of his behavior. My aim was to support their efforts to help him through difficult moments, so that he would learn to manage them himself. The progress was slow but steady, and he was increasingly able to tolerate social situations that had been highly fraught.

After working with me for about six months, with visits once every four to six weeks that sometimes included Pete and others just Lisa and Joe, a spot opened up at the medical center for an evaluation comprised of standardized assessment tools for diagnosing autism.

At a visit with me following that evaluation, Pete's parents described a two-hour session, during which several unfamiliar people asked questions while Pete sat on his father's lap. Lisa had missed the appointment as her aging mother had a health emergency the same day. The doctor had explained to Joe that Pete was supposed to get comfortable, but that never happened. Just the opposite occurred as both Pete and his father became increasingly stressed. When one of the doctors, intending to do a physical exam, approached Pete to take his shoes off, he had a full meltdown, and soon after the visit came to an end. At a follow-up visit two weeks later that Joe and Lisa both attended, they were handed the diagnosis of autism, and given a prescription for applied behavioral analysis (ABA), a method of treatment that focuses exclusively on behavior.

Both parents found the evaluation deeply unsettling. While Lisa appreciated her pediatrician's reassurance that Pete was "fine," it did not resonate with her experience of multiple parking lot meltdowns on the way to birthday parties and scenes of her dripping wet, hysterical son's begging not to do swim lessons with the other kids. But the diagnosis of autism also felt wrong, unless, as she said, "autism is so broadly defined that it becomes meaningless." She was caught between a wish to have an answer, and with it, the quick fix of what to do, and a wish to have time to understand him in the way that we had been working over the preceding months.

But finding the time was not the only challenge. Living with the uncertainty about what these current problems would look like as he grew up was very difficult, especially in the face of the certainty expressed by the "expert" at the medical center. Lisa feared that she was doing "nothing." "But it is not nothing," I said. "You are facing the sadness you feel that things are not easy for Pete." The tears began to flow. She was mourning the loss of the child for whom life went smoothly, the child she imagined. This mourning, as we saw in the preceding chapter, is an essential step toward the kind of presence needed to support Pete.

A graduate student at Massachusetts Institute of Technology highlights the subjective nature of the process of autism diagnosis in a fascinating study. He reviewed records from three clinics established specifically for evaluation of autism spectrum disorder. At two centers the rate of diagnosis was around 35 percent while at a third the rate was 65 percent. A news release about the study explains that the rates, even when other factors such as race, environment, and parent's education were accounted for, persisted over time. But perhaps most interesting, when doctors moved from one clinic to another, their rates of diagnosis changed to match that of the clinic. The study's author suggests, based on his extensive interviews and observations, that the differing rates were related to what he called "imprinting," or the influence of the different perspectives of "autism experts" who taught the doctors and directed the clinic. One emphasized the subtlety of signs of autism, encouraging staff to make the diagnosis, and the other conveyed his belief that autism can mimic other conditions, leading staff to be more cautious in handing out the diagnosis.

As we saw with Pete, once the purpose of the evaluation is to answer the question, "Does he or does he not have autism?" the possibility of exploration of the complexity of a child's experience is already limited. Referring to a recent trend to reframe the symptoms of autism as anxiety disorder, one pediatrician colleague described a kind of "aha" moment, saying excitedly, "Now I see that many of those kids diagnosed with autism really have anxiety disorder!" But both diagnostic labels may be similarly limiting.

At the end of the news release about the study, the author raises the question of how we "get at the truth" regarding autism diagnosis. This word resonated for me as an example of a search for certainty in situations of uncertainty. There is no "truth" for the diagnosis of autism or, for that matter, any other *DSM*-defined "mental disorders," all of which are based on subjective assessments of behavior or "symptoms."

The truth lies in our humanity, in the intricate interplay between biology and environment. It lies in the stories we tell and the meaning we make of our experience. The search for the truth requires patience, and protecting space and time to listen to those stories, in all their richness and complexity.

In my work with Pete and his parents I drew on my knowledge of the extensive research showing how parents pave a path to healthy development by reflecting on the meaning of behavior in just the way Pete's parents had been doing in our work together. I said to Lisa as she grappled with the lack of time, and the feeling that she was "doing nothing," that for Pete, what was most important for these early years was his parents' full presence through the difficult moments—the offer of containment and safety when he felt out of control. I was hopeful that by offering Joe and Lisa the opportunity to be heard and supported in this way, I would fortify them in their efforts to listen to Pete, to help him develop resilience in the face of his particular vulnerabilities. Rather than fruitlessly searching for "the truth," in tolerating uncertainty they were supporting the gradual development of his "true self."

The Danger of Certainty

For eighteen-year-old Mara, whose life was cut short, alone behind the wheel of her demolished car and with a blood alcohol level well above 0.08, the certainty of psychiatric diagnosis may have had deadly consequences. I met her mother Sally years after this event, when she had thrown her grief into work on prevention. To give meaning to this senseless loss, she wanted to do what she could to prevent this kind of outcome for others. She told me her story.

Mara had been treated for many years for ADHD. Now Sally was taking a long, hard look at her daughter's history and trying to make sense of her descent into substance abuse that led to this final tragic demise. Many doctors over the years had assured her that treatment of ADHD led to a decrease in substance abuse.

Mara was the youngest of three girls. Where her two older sisters excelled in school, she was "flighty." Even when she was as young as three, the rest of the family would get frustrated with her when she got easily distracted when asked to do a simple task like put on her shoes. In a busy household there was a lot of negative attention directed at Mara.

But in this time of careful and at times agonizing reflection, Sally acknowledged that Mara had been very curious and creative as well. She "noticed everything." At age five she was uncharacteristically quiet and attentive at a classical music concert, surprising her parents by identifying the individual instruments. But in a family of high academic achievers, when in first grade she lagged behind in learning to read, they took her to her pediatrician, who diagnosed ADHD and put her on stimulant medication.

Her doctors had seen it as a straightforward problem, no different from food allergies or diabetes: Mara had ADHD, so they gave her medication to treat it. The medication did have a remarkable effect on her ability to focus, from the first dose. But as the demands of school increased, the visits to the doctor consisted of changing dosages and formulas. Sally's heart ached as she recalled visits to the pediatrician where she spoke openly in front of Mara about her as "unmotivated" or even "lazy." Sally wondered whether the exclusive focus on Mara's dose of medication and her ability to get her homework done—they had added an evening dose when she started middle school and the academic challenges increased—had distracted them from appreciating Mara's individuality and from understanding her needs.

In this difficult conversation that Sally was determined to pursue, she came to see that Mara's inattentive behavior might have been connected to her creativity. She just experienced the world differently. In a soft voice that belied cries of agony, Sally wondered whether the firm, demanding parenting style that had been so effective with their first two was perhaps not ideal for Mara.

Once she felt comfortable telling me her story, other relevant information emerged. When Mara, an unplanned third child, was two years old, Sally became seriously ill. By the time Mara entered kindergarten Sally was well again. But during those early years she had not been able to give this active, sensitive toddler the attention she needed. In contrast, the two older girls had been a source of help and support. Her time and attention gravitated naturally to them. When Mara was evaluated for ADHD by her pediatrician, this part of the story, a difficult chapter they all wished to forget, never came up. Now Sally wondered whether Mara's "problem behavior" had been, at least in part, an effort to connect and get her mother's attention. She had heard people speak of ADHD as a deficit not of the child's ability to pay attention, but of the parents' attention to their child.

She had been doing her best for Mara. But perhaps she, the rest of the family, as well as the doctors who had treated Mara, hadn't really been listening to Mara. As the focus of her visits to the doctor became almost exclusively on the dose of medication and her academic performance, perhaps her "true self" got lost.

Reluctantly, Sally now shared with me a longstanding family history of covert substance abuse. She suspected that the pressure of the college application process was "the beginning of the end." Mara began drinking. In keeping with the family tradition, she was able to keep this fact well hidden from her parents.

Sally is not alone. A long-term follow-up study into adulthood of children diagnosed with ADHD shows not only a persistence of symptoms in one third of patients, but also a three times higher likelihood of what is termed comorbidity (substance abuse and other psychiatric diagnoses). In this study, the group of children diagnosed with ADHD had nearly five times higher risk of suicide than in a matched group without the diagnosis. Three percent were in prison. It is likely that parents, whose children were diagnosed with ADHD and have met tragic ends, struggle with questions similar to those Sally is facing.

The authors of that study, funded in part by McNeil Consumer and Specialty Pharmaceuticals, makers of Concerta (a popular drug for treatment of ADHD), concluded that ADHD is a chronic illness that requires lifelong treatment to avoid such dire outcomes. But there is a completely different way to interpret these findings. Could it be that the poor long-term outcomes are the result of not treating the problem properly in the first place? As we have seen, the standard of care in treatment is behavior therapy and medication, both of which attempt to change behavior without discovering its meaning. Had there been time and space to deconstruct the multiple factors contributing to the behavior in each child, would there have been opportunity to lead development toward a different, healthier path? Perhaps it is the silencing, the unheard stories, of families like Mara's, which leads so many to get worse rather than better.

A longing for certainty may grow out of helplessness and fear. When we struggle alone, an "expert" who offers the "answer" has powerful appeal. It takes courage for both parents and professionals to say, "I don't know." Not knowing opens the opportunity for saying, "I wonder," or "I'm curious," along with "Let's figure it out together." In being heard and understood a person can find both courage and confidence to tolerate uncertainty.

I came across a beautiful expression of the value of uncertainty in a very different context. In an article, "The Dangers of Certainty," Simon Critchley, a professor of philosophy at the New School, describes being profoundly influenced by the 1973 BBC documentary series *The Ascent of Man*, hosted by Dr. Jacob Bronowski.

Discussing Heisenberg's uncertainty principle, Bronowski, says Critchley, spoke of "a certain *toleration* of uncertainty. . . . We encounter other people across a gray area of negotiation and approximation. Such is the business of listening and the back and forth of conversation and social interaction."

Critchley continues: "As [Bronowski] eloquently put it, 'Human knowledge is personal and responsible, an unending adventure at the edge of uncertainty. The relationship between humans and nature and humans and other humans can take place only within a certain play of tolerance. Insisting on certainty, by contrast, leads ineluctably to arrogance and dogma based on ignorance.'"

Winnicott's good-enough mother offers the original experience of uncertainty. When she listens to her baby, not always "getting" what her baby is communicating, but taking the time to figure things out when she is off the mark, she is paving the way for social adaptation and the tolerant uncertainty inherent in all social interaction.

Finding the Right Words

"I meant what I said and I said what I meant . . . An elephant's faithful one-hundred percent." In Dr. Seuss's book *Horton Hatches the Egg,* Horton repeatedly recites these well-recognized words in his role as a kind of surrogate mother. He endures much hardship, including humiliation, weather disasters, and attacks by hunters, while sitting on the egg of his friend Mayzie the bird, waiting for it to hatch. With this powerful declaration of commitment to his promise, Horton tells us that he knows himself. Offering a kind of metaphor for parenting, Horton shows that when we know ourselves, we can stand by our children through the inevitable hardships of life.

Both children and parents find themselves through being heard. When parents hold a baby, not only with their body, but also with their voice and words, connecting feelings with language, the child's true self begins to take shape. Throughout our lives, the experience of being heard and understood echoes that original experience. A child's "problem behavior" represents big feelings, whether of anger, frustration, fear, anxiety, or sadness, that are out of control and not connected to words. As adults, especially as parents, we may also be flooded with emotions that get the better of us, without knowing why. When someone listens to us, we have a chance to connect the feelings with words, to make sense of our experience. The search for the right words is the search for the true self. When, like Horton, we can say what we mean and mean what we say, we find ourselves. In turn, we help our children to find themselves. Most important, when we know ourselves, we can listen to others.

For children and for parents, struggling, or the Buddhist no-tion of "ordinary suffering," is an inevitable part of development, not something to be diagnosed, managed, or medicated away. When we protect time and space to listen, for telling stories, for finding meaning, we have the opportunity to help our children and ourselves to move forward through healing toward growth and resilience.

Unless we make listening a priority, in families and in our health-care system, we risk not only a worsening epidemic of mental illness with its concurrent social ills, but also a legion of lost opportunities.

If instead, starting in the earliest weeks, months, and years of life, we consistently protect time and space for listening, both par-ents and professionals can foster a resilient generation in touch with their true selves. We could see an intergenerational transmis-sion of compassion, raising individuals who, in turn, have the abil-ity, like Horton, to offer their full presence and caring. By restoring a place for simply listening, we have every reason for hope.

Acknowledgments

First and foremost I would like to acknowledge the children and families who have given me the privilege of caring for them over many years of practice. Thanks to the efforts of my wonderful colleagues Michael Jellinek and Howard King, I have had the opportunity in recent years to listen to numerous stories of very young children and their families.

The faculty and fellows of the UMass Boston Infant-Parent Mental Health Post-Graduate Certificate Program provided, and continue to provide, invaluable ideas, support, inspiration, and friendship. Spending time in their presence always fortifies me to move forward, even at times when it feels that I am swimming against the tide.

I would also like to thank the faculty of the Berkshire Psychoanalytic Institute. When I began studying there in 2004, they opened my mind to a new way to think about and make sense of what I was observing every day in my pediatric practice.

I am indebted to my thoughtful, kind, and extremely patient agent, Lisa Adams, who read and revised countless versions. She stuck with me from the first moment, when this book was a kernel of its current form.

With my brilliant editor Merloyd Lawrence, I experienced a number of invaluable cycles of disruption and repair until we got to the place where the book she envisioned and the one I wanted to write were one and the same. I am thankful for her support and persistence. She did not let up until I had communicated exactly what I meant to say.

I am most grateful for my husband, who has strongly and consistently supported my off-the-beaten-path career trajectory, and for my children, who continue to be my greatest teachers, while bringing me endless joy and pride as I watch them grow into young adults.

And last, I would like to thank my parents. Even though I did not end up writing a book about my father, he is present throughout the pages of this one. My parents embody the qualities of hope and resilience. Just as my father's loss lives in me, so does his optimism. He lives life forward, with strength, engagement, and enthusiasm. I have inherited from him the drive and persistence to right a wrong, and to use my voice to give voice to the silenced children.

Notes

Introduction: The Power of Listening

xiv   *Listening to a child in this way:* P. Fonagy, G. Gergely, E. Jurist, and M. Target, *Affect Regulation, Mentalization and the Development of the Self* (New York: Other Press, 2002).

        E. L. Jurist, A. Slade, and S. Bergner, eds., *Mind to Mind: Infant Research, Neuroscience, and Psychoanalysis* (New York: Other Press, 2008).

        J. G. Allen, P. Fonagy, and A. W. Bateman, eds., *Mentalizing in Clinical Practice* (Washington, DC/London: American Psychiatric Publishing, 2008).

        Fredric N. Busch, ed., *Mentalization: Theoretical Considerations, Research Findings and Clinical Implications* (New York: Analytic Press, 2008).

        L. Mayes, P. Fonagy, and M. Target, eds., *Developmental Science and Psychoanalysis* (London: Karnac Books, 2007).

xiv   *I have shortened in my work:* C. M. Gold, *Keeping Your Child in Mind: Overcoming Defiance, Tantrums, and other Everyday Behavior Problems by Seeing the World Through Your Child's Eyes* (Boston: Da Capo Press, 2011).

xiv   *Similar concepts of listening:* T. N. Hanh, *The Heart of the Buddha's Teaching: Transforming Suffering into Peace, Joy, and Liberation* (New York: Broadway Books, 1998), 86–88.

xv   *Recent statistics indicate that diagnosis of ADHD:* Susanna N. Visser, MS, DrPH, "Diagnostic Experiences of Children with Attention-Deficit/Hyperactivity Disorder," Centers for Disease Control and Prevention National Health Statistics Report Number 81, September 3, 2015.

xv   *The diagnosis of autism rose:* "CDC Estimates 1 in 68 Children Has Been Identified with Autism Spectrum Disorder," Centers for Disease Control and Prevention, March 27, 2014, http://www.cdc.gov/media/releases/2014/p0327 -autism-spectrum-disorder.html.

xv   *A 4,000 percent rise in diagnosis of childhood bipolar disorder:* C. Moreno et al., "National Trends in the Outpatient Diagnosis and Treatment of Bipolar Disorder in Youth," *Archives of General Psychiatry* 64, no. 9 (September 2007): 1032–39.

xv   *A close to 500 percent increase:* D. J. Safer et al., "Increased Methylphenidate

Usage for Attention Deficit Disorder in the 1990s," *Pediatrics* 98 (December 1996): 1084–88.

"Key Findings: Trends in the Parent-Report of Health Care Provider-Diagnosis and Medication Treatment for ADHD: United States, 2003–2011," Centers for Disease Control and Prevention, http://www.cdc.gov/ncbddd/adhd/features/key-findings-adhd72013.html.

xvi   *But psychoanalyst Sally Provence:* Fredric N. Busch, ed., *Mentalization: Theoretical Considerations, Research Findings and Clinical Implications* (New York: Analytic Press, 2008), 225.

xviii   *Charles Darwin, in a work of great observation:* Charles Darwin, *The Expression of the Emotions in Man and Animals* (New York: Penguin Classics, 1890, 2009).

xxiii   *When a recent study, widely publicized:* N. Zucker et al., "Psychological and Psychosocial Impairment in Preschoolers with Selective Eating," *Pediatrics*, 36, no. 3 (September 2015).

xxiii   *with such headlines as:* Rachel Rabkin Peachman, "Picky Eating in Children Linked to Anxiety, Depression, and ADHD," *New York Times*, August 3, 2015.

xxiv   *"Many of us have lost our capacity:* T. N. Hanh, *The Heart of the Buddha's Teaching: Transforming Suffering into Peace, Joy, and Liberation* (New York: Broadway Books, 1998), 88.

Chapter 1: On (Not) Giving Advice

3   *"No theory is acceptable:* D. W. Winnicott, "Ego Distortions in Terms of True and False Self," in *The Maturational Process and the Facilitating Environment* (New York: International Universities Press, 1965), 148.

3   *In an essay ironically titled:* D. W. Winnicott, *Winnicott on the Child* (Cambridge, MA: Perseus Publishing, 2002), 193–201.

4   *Journalist Jennifer Senior describes how:* Jennifer Senior, *All Joy and No Fun: The Paradox of Modern Parenthood* (New York: Harper Collins, 2014).

Jennifer Senior, "For Parents Happiness Is a Very High Bar," TED Talk, filmed March 2014, http://www.ted.com/talks/jennifer_senior_for_parents_happiness_is_a_very_high_bar.

5   *The "good-enough" mother (not necessarily the infant's own mother):* D. W. Winnicott, *Playing and Reality* (London and New York: Routledge Classics, 2005), 14.

6   *The story of a human being:* D. W. Winnicott, *The Child, the Family and the Outside World* (New York: Perseus Publishing, 1964), 86.

6   *another central concept of Winnicott's:* D. W. Winnicott "Ego Distortions in Terms of True and False Self," in *The Maturational Process and the Facilitating Environment* (New York: International Universities Press, 1965), 140–52.

7   *In his wise book:* Andrew Solomon, *Far from the Tree: Parents, Children, and the Search for Identity* (New York: Scribner, 2012).

11   *He defines the concept as:* P. Fonagy and E. Allison, "The Role of Mentalizing and Epistemic Trust in the Therapeutic Relationship," *Psychotherapy* 51, no. 3 (2014): 373.

12   *John Bowlby was among the first:* J. Bowlby, *A Secure Base: Parent-Child Attachment and Healthy Human Development* (New York: Basic Books, 1988).

12   *Capturing the essence of:* J. Bowlby, *A Secure Base: Parent-Child Attachment and Healthy Human Development* (New York: Basic Books, 1988), 82.

Chapter 2: Listening Devalued

14   *A 2013 CDC:* Bruce S. Jonas et al., "Psychotropic Medication Use Among Adolescents: United States, 2005–2010," NCHS Data Brief Number 135, December 2013, http://www.cdc.gov/nchs/data/databriefs/db135.htm.

14   *Marcia Angell, former editor:* Marcia Angell, "The Illusions of Psychiatry," *New York Review of Books,* July 14, 2011.

15   *In my first book:* C. M. Gold, *Keeping Your Child in Mind: Overcoming Defiance, Tantrums, and other Everyday Behavior Problems by Seeing the World Through Your Child's Eyes* (Boston: Da Capo Press, 2011).

15   *The areas of the brain responsible for:* Allan Schore, *Affect Regulation and the Origin of the Self: The Neurobiology of Emotional Development* (New York: Psychology Press, 1994).

> Allan Schore, *Affect Regulation and Disorders of the Self* (New York: W. W. Norton & Company, 2003).
>
> Allan Schore, *Affect Regulation and Repair of the Self* (New York: W. W. Norton & Company, 2003).
>
> Daniel J. Siegel, *The Developing Mind: How Relationships and the Brain Interact to Shape Who We Are* (New York: Guilford Press, 1999).

16   *In a course she teaches:* Francine Lapides, MFT, clinical course "Keeping the Brain in Mind," Cape Cod Institute, 2010.

16   *A recent study documented:* J. N. Epstein, K. J. Kelleher, R. Baum, W. B. Brinkman, J. Peugh, W. Gardner, P. Lichtenstein, and J. Langberg, "Variability in ADHD Care in Community-Based Pediatrics," *Pediatrics* 134, no. 6 (December 2014): 1136–43.

21   *"If you ask questions you get answers:* Michael Balint, *The Doctor, His Patient and the Illness* (Madison, WI: International Universities Press, 1957), 133.

22   *"The discussion quickly revealed:* Ibid., 1.

22   *The very structure of the DSM:* *Diagnostic and Statistical Manual of Mental Disorders,* 5th ed. (New York: American Psychiatric Association, 2013).

22   *A recent publication by:* Philip R. Muskin, MD, *DSM-5 Self-Exam Questions: Test Questions for the Diagnostic Criteria,* American Psychiatric Association, 2014, 51.

23   *Psychologist Jonathan Shedler:* Jonathan Shedler, "Doublethink Diagnosis 2.0: A Psychiatric Diagnosis Cannot Be the 'Cause' of Anything," *Psychologically Minded* 01 (blog), October 2013, https://www.psychologytoday.com/blog/psychologically-minded/2013"10/doublethink-diagnosis-20.

23   *While studying for my recertification exam:* American Academy of Pediatrics, *2014 PREP Self-Assessment* Q-48 C-146.

26   *In one of the novel's most famous quotes:* Harper Lee, *To Kill a Mockingbird* (New York: Harper Collins, 2010), 48.

26   *Psychoanalyst Peter Fonagy argues:* Fredric N. Busch, ed., *Mentalization: The-oretical Considerations, Research Findings and Clinical Implications* (New York: Analytic Press, 2008), 5.

26   *in a way similar to John Bowlby's representation:* John Bowlby, *Attachment* (New York: Basic Books, 1982).

Chapter 3: Listening to Babies

34   *Recent longitudinal research:* R. Hyde, M. O'Callaghan, W. Bor, G. Williams, and J. Najman, "Long-term Outcomes of Infant Behavioral Dysregulation," *Pediatrics* 130, no. 5 (November 2012).

35   *I was fortunate to be able to:* Infant-Parent Mental Health Fellowship/Post-graduate Certificate Program University of Massachusetts Boston, https://www.umb.edu/academics/cla/psychology/professional_development/infant-parent-mental-health.

36   *The work of British researchers:* L. Murray and P. Cooper, eds., *Postpartum Depression and Child Development* (New York: Guilford Press, 1997).

          L. Murray, A. Arteche, P. Fearon, S. Halligan, I. Goodyer, and P. Cooper, "Maternal Postnatal Depression and the Development of Depression in Offspring up to 16 Years of Age," *Journal of the American Academy of Child and Adolescent Psychiatry* 50, no. 5 (2011) 460–70.

36   *Ed Tronick's mutual regulation model:* Ed Tronick, *The Neurobehavioral and Social-Emotional Development of Infants and Children* (New York, London: W. W. Norton & Company, 2007).

          J. A. DiCorcia and E. Tronick, "Quotidian Resilience: Exploring Mecha-nisms That Drive Resilience from a Perspective of Everyday Stress and Coping," *Neuroscience and Biobehavioral Reviews* 35 (2011): 1593–1602.

36   *While I was already familiar with:* P. Fonagy, G. Gergely, E. Jurist, and M. Tar-get, *Affect Regulation, Mentalization and the Development of the Self* (New York: Other Press, 2002).

36   *recent evidence that certain medications:* M. L. Hudak and R. C. Tan, "Neona-tal Drug Withdrawal," *Pediatrics* 129, no. 2 (2012): e540–e560.

37   *in an equally important evolutionary adaptation:* Kate Wong, "Why Humans Give Birth to Helpless Babies," *Scientific American* (blog post), August 28, 2012, http://blogs.scientificamerican.com/observations/why-humans-give-birth-to-helpless-babies/.

37   *These two adaptations come together:* J. Ronald Lally, "The Human Brain's Need for a 'Social Womb' During Infancy," For Our Babies, April 2014, http://forourbabies.org/wp-content/uploads/2014/04/The-Human-Brains-Need-for-a-Social-WombFINALApril2014.pdf.

38   *He referred to this kind of completely consuming care:* D. W. Winnicott, "Pri-mary Maternal Preoccupation," in *Through Pediatrics to Psychoanalysis* (New York: Basic Books, 1975), 300–305.

38   *Research into the neurobiological and genetic:* L. Mayes, J. E. Swain, and J. F. Leckman, "Parental Attachment Systems: Neural Circuits, Genes, and Ex-periential Contributions to Parental Engagement," *Clinical Neuroscience Re-search* 4 (2005): 301–13.

38   *As Linda Mayes of the Yale Child Study Center:* L. Mayes, P. Fonagy, and M. Target, eds., *Developmental Science and Psychoanalysis* (London: Karnac Books, 2007), 92.

38   *In a beautiful film: the connected baby:* A film conversation by Suzanne Zeedyk and Jonathan Robertson.

39   *In the words of Winnicott biographer:* Adam Phillips, *Winnicott* (Cambridge, MA: Harvard University Press, 1988), 128.

39   *As Winnicott wisely observes:* D. W. Winnicott, "The Theory of the Parent-Infant Relationship," in *The Maturational Process and the Facilitating Environment* (New York: International Universities Press, 1965), 49.

40   *Then, one day, they find:* D. W. Winnicott, "The Ordinary Devoted Mother" in *Winnicott on the Child* (Cambridge, MA: Perseus Publishing, 2002), 12.

42   *The book is James Agee's:* James Agee, *A Death in the Family* (New York: Penguin Books, 2008), 27.

44   *as recently recommended by the US Preventive Services Task Force:* "Depression in Adults Screening," US Preventive Task Force Services, August 2015, http://www.uspreventiveservicestaskforce.org/Page/Document/draft -recommendation-statement115/depression-in-adults-screening1.

46   *Working with mother-baby pairs:* Elizabeth Werner et al., "PREPP: Postpartum Depression Prevention Through the Mother–Infant Dyad," *Archives of Women's Mental Health* (August 2, 2015).

50   *development of the Neonatal Behavioral Assessment Scale:* T. B. Brazelton and J. K. Nugent, *Neonatal Behavioral Assessment Scale,* 4th ed. (London: Mac Keith Press, 2011).

50   *The NBO, developed by psychologist J. Kevin Nugent:* J. K. Nugent, C. Keefer, S. Minear, L. C. Johnson, and Y. Blanchard, *Understanding Newborn Behavior & Early Relationships: The Newborn Behavioral Observation (NBO) System Handbook* (Baltimore, MD: Paul H. Brookes Publishing, 2007).

50   *One study showed a significant decrease:* J. Kevin Nugent et al., "The Effects of an Infant-Focused Relationship-Based Hospital and Home Visiting Intervention on Reducing Symptoms of Postpartum Maternal Depression," *Infants and Young Children* 27, no. 4 (2014): 292–304.

51   *Projection can take many complex forms:* S. H. Fraiberg, E. Adelson, et al., "Ghosts in the Nursery: A Psychoanalytic Approach to the Problem of Impaired Mother-Infant Relationships," *Journal of the American Academy of Child and Adolescent Psychiatry* 14 (1975): 387–422.

52   *An ongoing study at Austen Riggs Center:* Donna Elmendorf, personal communication, June 2015.

55   *Research of Pulitzer Prize–winning economist:* James Heckman, "Schools, Skills and Synapses," *Economic Inquiry* 46, no. 3 (2008): 289.

56   *suggested to a pediatrician colleague:* Harwood Egan, personal communication, May 2014.

56   *videotape, when parents, together with a clinician:* Miriam Steele et al., "Looking from the Outside In: The Use of Video in Attachment-Based Interventions, *Attachment & Human Development* 16, no. 4 (2014), 402–15.

Chapter 4: Listening as Prevention

59   *A large long-term study sponsored by the CDC:* Centers for Disease Control and Prevention, "Injury Prevention & Control: Division of Violence Prevention," the ACE Study, May 13, 2014, http://www.cdc.gov/violenceprevention /acestudy/.

60   *In a fascinating review of this complex field:* M. Kundakovic and F. Champagne, "Early Life Experience, Epigenetics, and the Developing Brain," *Neuropsychopharmacology REVIEWS* 40 (2015): 141–53.

60   *John Green and colleagues:* J. Green et al., "Parent-Mediated Intervention Versus No Intervention for Infants at High Risk of Autism: A Parallel, Single-Blind, Randomized Trial," *Lancet Psychiatry* 2, no. 2 (2015): 133–40.

63   *A recent article in the journal* Pediatrics: E. K. Balog, J. L. Hanson, and G. S. Blaschke, "Teaching the Essentials of 'Well-Child Care': Inspiring Proficiency and Passion," *Pediatrics* 34, no. 2 (2014): 206–9.

63   *Touchpoints theory and programs:* T. Berry Brazelton and Joshua Sparrow, *Touchpoints: Birth to Three: Your Child's Emotional and Behavioral Development* (Cambridge MA: Da Capo Press, 2006).

64   *about the first year of life:* Yudhijit Bhattacharjee, "The First Year," *National Geographic,* January 2015.

69   *Psychiatrist Bruce Perry has developed:* Laurie MacKinnon, "The Neurosequential Model of Therapeutics: An Interview with Bruce Perry," *Australian and New Zealand Journal of Family Therapy* 33, no. 3 (2012): 210–18.

Chapter 5: Time and Space for Listening

73   *In his book* The Examined Life: Stephen Grosz, *The Examined Life: How We Lose Ourselves and Find Ourselves* (New York: W. W. Norton & Company, 2013), 21.

74   *In her book* Overwhelmed: Brigid Schulte, *Overwhelmed: Work, Love, and Play When No One Has the Time* (New York: Picador, 2014).

78   *Research by Stephen Porges:* Stephen Porges, *The Polyvagal Theory: Neurophysiologic Foundations of Emotions, Attachment, Communication and Self-regulation* (New York, W. W. Norton & Company, 2011).

79   *In his introduction to Porges's book:* Ibid., xvi.

80   *"It is in playing and only in playing:* D. W. Winnicott, *Playing and Reality* (London and New York: Routledge Classics, 2005), 73.

80   *Later in the same work:* Ibid., 86.

80   *Dancing Lessons, a play recently premiered:* Mark St. Germain, *Dancing Lessons,* Dramatist's Play Service, Inc., 2015.

81   *editor M. Gerard Fromm shares a vignette:* M. Gerard Fromm, ed., *A Spirit That Impels: Play, Creativity, and Psychoanalysis* (London: Karnac Books, 2014), xx.

83   *Winnicott writes, "In these highly specialized conditions:* D. W. Winnicott, *Playing and Reality* (London and New York: Routledge Classics, 2005), 76.

85   *One group leader articulated this idea:* Divya Kumar, "It's Not Just You: Creating Safe Spaces for Moms to Share," *MotherWoman Supporting and Empowering*

Mothers (blog), February 17, 2015, http://www.huffingtonpost.com/mother woman/its-not-just-you-creating_b_6349018.html.

85   *The value of the physical space:* Bright Spaces® A Special Place for Children, Bright Horizons Foundation for Children, http://www.brighthorizons foundation.org/what-we-do/bright-spaces/.

86   *Children's book on toilet training:* C. M. Gold, "A Parents' Guide to Toilet Training," in *Potty Palooza: A Step-by-Step Guide to Using a Potty*, by Rachel Gordon (New York: Workman Publishing, 2013).

94   *A recent study showed:* Danielle Ofri, "Adventures in Prior Authorization," *New York Times*, August 3, 2014.

95   *Howard King, runs a wonderful program:* Children's Emotional Healthlink 2015, http://www.cehl.org/.

97   *The Healthy Steps^SM program, developed by Margot Kaplan-Sanoff:* B. Zuckerman et al., "Healthy Steps: A Case Study of Innovation in Pediatric Practice" *Pediatrics* 114, no. 3 (September 2004).

Chapter 6: The Rush to Label and Medicate

101   *In the introductory chapter of his book:* Michael Balint, *The Doctor, His Patient and the Illness* (Madison, WI: International Universities Press, 1957), 1.

101   *An article about the placebo effect:* Danielle Ofri, "A Powerful Tool in the Doctor's Toolkit," Well, *New York Times* (blog), August 15, 2013, http://well .blogs.nytimes.com/2013/08/15/a-powerful-tool-in-the-doctors-toolkit/.

102   *Serious mental health problems in the college community:* American Psychological Association, "College Students' Mental Health Is a Growing Concern, Survey Finds," *Monitor on Psychology* 44, no. 6 (June 2013), http://www.apa .org/monitor/2013/06/college-students.aspx.

102   *A survey of close to two thousand people:* John Read et al., "Adverse Emotional and Interpersonal Effects Reported by 1829 New Zealanders While Taking Antidepressants," *Psychiatry Research* 216, no. 1 (April 30 2014): 67–73.

102   *A recent report showed that close to 1 in 3:* Center for the Study of Collegiate Mental Health, 2009 pilot study: executive summary, April 2009, 11, http:// ccmh.psu.edu/wp-content/uploads/sites/3058/2014/07/2009_CCMH _Report.pdf.

102   *At a conference exploring this escalating use:* M. G. Fromm, "The Escalating Use of Medication by College Students: What Are They Telling Us, What Are We Telling them?" in *Pharmacological Treatment of College Students with Psychological Problems*, eds. Leighton C. Whitaker and Stewart E. Cooper (New York: Routledge, 2007), 30.

103   *Patricia Wen, a Boston Globe reporter:* Patricia Wen, "The Other Welfare: A Legacy of Unintended Side Effects," *Boston Globe*, December 12, 2010, http://www.boston.com/news/local/massachusetts/articles/2010/12/12 /with_ssi_program_a_legacy_of_unintended_side_.

Patricia Wen, "Aid to Disabled Children Now Outstrips Welfare," *Boston Globe*, August 28, 2014, https://www.bostonglobe.com/metro/2014 /08/27/cash-distributed-under-ssi-for-children-now-exceeds-welfare /ekOpeSWTLJ00YId0CONFYI/story.html#.

105   *Multiple drugs (polypharmacy) are increasingly used:* Bruce Jancin, "Psychotropic Polypharmacy Widespread in Pediatric Primary Care," in *Pediatric Academic Societies*, May 4, 2015, http://www.pm360online.com/pas-psychotropic-poly pharmacy-widespread-in-pediatric-primary-care/.

105   *They are known to cause not only:* Lawrence Maayan, MD, and Christoph U. Correll, MD, "Weight Gain and Metabolic Risks Associated with Antipsychotic Medications in Children and Adolescents," *Journal of Child and Adolescent Psychopharmacology* 21, no. 6 (December 2011): 517–35.

105   *Despite the fact that no sleep medications:* "Trends in Medication Prescribing for Pediatric Sleep Difficulties in US Outpatient Settings," *Sleep* 30, no 8 (2007): 1013–1017.

107   *A recent study that received a lot:* Rebecca J. Scharf, MD, MPH, Ryan T. Demmer, PhD, MPH, Ellen J. Silver, PhD; and Ruth E. K. Stein, MD, "Nighttime Sleep Duration and Externalizing Behaviors of Preschool Children," *Journal of Developmental & Behavioral Pediatrics* 34, no. 6 (July/August 2013): 384–91.

110   *In a blog post:* Jane Ellen Stevens, "Pediatricians Screen Parents for ACEs to Improve Health of Babies," *ACEs Too High* (blog), August 3, 2015, http:// acestoohigh.com/2015/08/03/pediatricians-screen-parents-for-aces-to -improve-health-of-babies/.

112   *An alarming recent study showed that:* Mehmet Burcu, Julie Magno Zito, Aloysius Ibe, and Daniel J. Safer, "Atypical Antipsychotic Use Among Medicaid-Insured Children and Adolescents: Duration, Safety, and Monitoring Implications," *Journal of Child and Adolescent Psychopharmacology* 24, no. 3 (April 2014): 112–19.

112   *Given what we know about intergenerational transmission:* C. Zeanah and P. Zeanah, "Intergenerational Transmission of Maltreatment: Insights from Attachment Theory and Research," *Psychiatry: Interpersonal and Biological Processes* 52, no. 2 (1989).

113   *Psychologist Ed Tronick references:* Ed Tronick, "The Still-Face Experiment," YouTube, July 7, 2013, https://www.youtube.com/watch?v=C8ZTx1AEup4.

114   *Psychoanalyst Robert Furman offers an alternative:* Robert Furman, "Attention Deficit Hyperactivity Disorder: An Alternative Viewpoint," *Journal of Infant, Child, and Adolescent Psychotherapy* 2, no. 1 (2002).

116   *In the play and film* God of Carnage: Yasmina Reza, *God of Carnage*, Dramatist's Play Service, Inc., June 4, 2009.

117   *A recent study, one that supports:* K. D. Gadow et al., "Risperidone Added to Parent Training and Stimulant Medication: Effects on Attention-Deficit/ Hyperactivity Disorder, Oppositional Defiant Disorder, Conduct Disorder, and Peer Aggression," *Journal of the American Academy of Child and Adolescent Psychiatry* 53, no. 9 (2014): 948–59.

120   *For example, diagnosis of ADHD in children:* B. D. Fulton et al., "State Variation in Increased ADHD Prevalence: Links to NCLB School Accountability and State Medication Laws," October 1, 2015, http://ps.psychiatryonline .org/doi/abs/10.1176/appi.ps.201400145?journalCode=ps.

120   *The 2011 change in the AAP:* "ADHD: Clinical Practice Guideline for the Diagnosis, Evaluation, and Treatment of Attention-Deficit/Hyperactivity Disorder in Children and Adolescents," *Pediatrics* 128, no. 5 (November 2011).

120   *A report from the Department of Education:* The Editorial Board, "Giving Up on Four-Year-Olds," *New York Times*, March 26, 2014, http://www.nytimes.com/2014/03/27/opinion/giving-up-on-4-year-olds.html?_r=0.

121   *In one study, teachers were:* Walter S. Gilliam and Golan Shahar, "Preschool and Child Care Expulsion and Suspension: Rates and Predictors in One State," *Infants & Young Children* 19, no. 3 (July–Sep 2006): 228–45.

121   *Such a series of events:* Kelly Wallace, "The Handcuffed Boy Video: How to Discipline Children with ADHD," CNN, August 7, 2015, http://www.cnn.com/2015/08/06/health/disciplining-kids-with-adhd-handcuffed-boy/index.html.

121   *Jane Ellen Stevens writes about one such program:* Jane Ellen Stevens, *Lincoln High School in Walla Walla, WA, Tries New Approach to School Discipline—Suspensions Drop 85% ACES Too High News*, April 23, 2012, http://acestoohigh.com/2012/04/23/lincoln-high-school-in-walla-walla-wa-tries-new-approach-to-school-discipline-expulsions-drop-85/.

122   *in his new documentary* Paper Tigers: http://papertigersmovie.com/.

122   *In a blog post about his experience:* James Redford, "Can School Heal Children in Pain?" *Bright* (blog), June 1, 2015, https://medium.com/bright/can-school-heal-children-in-pain-d9ef3abb9176.

123   *As psychiatrist Bessel Van der Kolk writes:* Bessel Van der Kolk, *The Body Keeps Score: Brain, Mind, and Body in the Healing of Trauma* (New York: Viking, 2014), 352.

124   *there is evidence not only that:* Irene M. Loe, MD, and Heidi M. Feldman, MD, PHD, "Academic and Educational Outcomes of Children with ADHD," *Journal of Pediatric Psychology* 32, no. 6 (2007): 643–54.
        Katherine Sharpe, "The Smart-Pill Oversell: Evidence Is Mounting That Medication for ADHD Doesn't Make a Lasting Difference to School-work or Achievement," *Nature International Weekly Journal of Science* 506, no. 7487 (February 2014).

124   *ADHD symptoms do not go away:* William J. Barbaresi, MD, Robert C. Colligan, PhD, Amy L. Weaver, MS, Robert G. Voigt, MD, Jill M. Killian, BS, and Slavica K. Katusic, MD, "Mortality, ADHD, and Psychosocial Adversity in Adults with Childhood ADHD: A Prospective Study," *Pediatrics* 131, no. 4 (April 2013).

124   *The gold standard in ADHD treatment:* Peter S. Jensen et al., "Findings from the NIMH Multimodal Treatment Study of ADHD (MTA): Implications and Applications for Primary Care Providers," *Journal of Developmental and Behavioral Pediatrics* 22, no. 1 (February 2001).

124   *At the eight-year follow-up:* Brooke S. G. Molina, PhD, et al., "The MTA at 8 Years: Prospective Follow-up of Children Treated for Combined-Type ADHD in a Multisite Study," *Journal of the American Academy of Child and Adolescent Psychiatry* 48, no. 5 (2009): 484–500.

125   *A long-term follow-up study of ADHD diagnosed in preschool:* Mark Riddle et

al., "The Preschool Attention-Deficit/Hyperactivity Disorder Treatment Study (PATS) 6-Year Follow-Up," *Journal of the American Academy of Child and Adolescent Psychiatry* 52, no. 3 (March 2013): 264–78.

127 *The study from a group of physicians:* F. T. Bourgeois et al., "Premarket Safety and Efficacy Studies for ADHD Medications in Children," *PLOS ONE* (July 9, 2014), http://journals.plos.org/plosone/article?id=10.1371/journal.pone .0102249.

127 *"Reviewers were mainly concerned that:* Florence Bourgeois, MD, MPH, personal communication, September 2014.

Chapter 7: Prejudice Against Children

129 *publication of her book* Childism; Elisabeth Young-Bruehl, *Childism: Confronting Prejudice Against Children* (New Haven, CT: Yale University Press, 2012).

129 *She defines* childism *as:* Ibid., 37.

130 *She writes of "a childism of the sort:* Ibid., 254.

131 *Whole books are written about:* Russell A. Barkley and Christine M. Benton, *Your Defiant Child: 8 Steps to Better Behavior* (New York: Guilford Press, 2013).

133 *A dramatic example is the* Defiant Requiem: http://www.defiantrequiem.org /thedocumentary.

133 *In a* Time *magazine piece:* D. J. Siegel and T. Payne Bryson, "Time-Outs Are Hurting Your Child," *Time*, September 23, 2014, http://time.com/3404701 /discipline-time-out-is-not-good/.

133 *following the release of his new book:* D. J. Siegel and T. Payne Bryson, *No-Drama Discipline: The Whole-Brain Way to Calm the Chaos and Nurture Your Child's Developing Mind*, (New York: Bantam Books, 2014).

135 *an entire symposium on the subject:* "Punishing a Child Is Effective If Done Correctly," American Psychological Association, August 6, 2015, http:// www.apa.org/news/press/releases/2015/08/punishing-child.aspx.

137 *Young-Bruehl compares the situation in our country:* Elisabeth Young-Bruehl, *Childism: Confronting Prejudice Against Children* (New Haven, CT: Yale University Press, 2012), 138.

137 *She astutely observes:* Ibid., 270.

137 *policy statement of the American Academy of Pediatrics:* Andrew Garner et al., "Early Childhood Adversity, Toxic Stress, and the Role of the Pediatrician: Translating Developmental Science into Lifelong Health," *Pediatrics* 121, no. 1 (2012): e224–e231.

138 *A powerful documentary film:* http://webspecial.mercurynews.com/drugged kids/.

139 *Elegant and compelling research:* Martin Teicher, MD, PhD, and Jacqueline Samson, PhD, "Childhood Maltreatment and Psychopathology: A Case for Ecophenotypic Variants as Clinically and Neurobiologically Distinct Subtypes," *American Journal of Psychiatry* 170, no. 10 (October 1, 2013).

140 *whose work is featured in Young-Bruehl's book:* Elisabeth Young-Bruehl, *Childism: Confronting Prejudice Against Children* (New Haven, CT: Yale University Press, 2012), 275–80.

Chapter 8: Listening to the Body: Paths to Healing

143   *In the documentary:* http://webspecial.mercurynews.com/druggedkids/.

144   *Pediatrician T. Berry Brazelton:* T. B. Brazelton and J. K. Nugent *Neonatal Behavioral Assessment Scale,* 4th ed. (London: Mac Keith Press, 2011).

146   *a parent teaches this essential skill to a child. Zeedyk writes:* Suzanne Zeedyk, "On the Value of Emotional Regulation, aka 'Keeping Your Feelings in Check," *The Science of Human Connection* (blog), December 27, 2011, http://suzanne zeedyk.co.uk/wp2/2011/12/27/on-the-value-of-emotional-regulation-aka -keeping-your-feelings-in-check/.

146   *described in a 2009 article:* David Dobbs, "The Science of Success," *Atlantic,* December 2009, http://www.theatlantic.com/magazine/archive/2009/12/the -science-of-success/307761/.

147   *Offering evidence to support this theory:* Timothy B. Nguyen, Jane M. Gunn, Maria Potiriadis, Ian P. Everall, and Chad A. Bousman, "Serotonin Transporter Polymorphism (*5HTTLPR*), Severe Childhood Abuse and Depressive Symptom Trajectories in Adulthood," *British Journal of Psychiatry Open* 1, no. 1 (September 2015): 104–9.

147   *In a press release, the lead author:* "Gene Tied to Adult Depression After Childhood Abuse," HealthDay, September 24, 2015, http://consumer.healthday .com/mental-health-information-25/depression-news-176/gene-tied-to-adult -depression-after-childhood-abuse-703465.html.

147   *In a beautiful example:* Philip Schultz, *My Dyslexia* (New York: W. W. Norton, 2011).

149   *Of the "holding environment" that offers:* D. W. Winnicott, "The Theory of the Parent-Infant Relationship," in *The Maturational Process and the Facilitating Environment* (New York: International Universities Press, 1965), 49.

149   *Controversy swirls around the question:* Suzanne Allard Levingston, "The Debate over Sensory Processing Disorder: Are Some Kids Really 'Out of Sync'?" Health and Science, *Washington Post,* May 12 2014,http://www.washington post.com/national/health-science/the-debate-over-sensory-processing -disorder-are-some-kids-really-out-of-sync/2014/05/12/fca2d338-d521–11e3 –8a78–8fe50322a72c_story.html.

152   *He developed a model of assessment:* "DIR® and the DIRFloortime® Approach," ICDL Interdisciplinary Council on Development and Learning, http://www.icdl.com/DIR.

152   *DIR Floortime™ is a form of treatment:* Jean Mercer, "Examining DIR/Floortime™ as a Treatment for Children with Autism Spectrum Disorders: A Review of Research and Theory," *Research on Social Work Practice,* May 24, 2015.

153   *A recent policy statement:* American Academy of Pediatrics, policy statement, "Sensory Integration Therapies for Children with Developmental and Behavioral Disorders," *Pediatrics* online, May 28, 2012, http://pediatrics .aappublications.org/content/pediatrics/early/2012/05/23/peds.2012–0876. full.pdf.

153   *Consider this poignant description:* Daphne Merkin, "A Journey Through Darkness—My Life with Chronic Depression," *New York Times Magazine,* May 6, 2009.

155   *The Neurosequential Model of Therapeutics:* Laurie MacKinnon, "The Neurosequential Model of Therapeutics: An Interview with Bruce Perry," *Australian and New Zealand Journal of Family Therapy* 33, no. 3 (2012): 210–18.

156   *Being outside, particularly in nature:* Gregory N. Bratman et al., "Nature Experience Reduces Rumination and Subgenual Prefrontal Cortex Activation," *Proceedings of the National Academy of Sciences* 12, no. 28 (July 14, 2015): 8567–72.

157   *Recent research exploring the role of exercise:* Matthew B. Pontifex et al., "Exercise Improves Behavioral, Neurocognitive, and Scholastic Performance in Children with ADHD," *Journal of Pediatrics* 162, no. 3 (March 2013): 543–51.

157   *In one study, children diagnosed with ADHD:* T. A. Hartanto, C. E. Krafft, A. M. Iosif, and J. B. Schweitzer, "A Trial-by-Trial Analysis Reveals More Intense Physical Activity Is Associated with Better Cognitive Control Performance in Attention-Deficit/Hyperactivity Disorder," *Child Neuropsychology* (June 10, 2015): 1–9.

157   *In a widely read article published in the* Washington Post: Valerie Strauss and Angela Hanscom, "Why So Many Kids Can't Sit Still in School Today," *Washington Post*, July 8, 2014, http://www.washingtonpost.com/blogs/answer-sheet/wp/2014/07/08/why-so-many-kids-cant-sit-still-in-school-today/.

158   *Infant massage, a well-known tool:* Caroline Zealey, "The Benefits of Infant Massage: A Critical Review," *Community Practitioner* 78, no. 3 (March 2005): 98–102.

159   *she produced an album for parents and babies:* Vered Benhorin, *Good Morning My Love: Songs to Bond You and Your* Baby, Jon Samson, CoCreative Music, October 23, 2012.

159   *I found the following on her website:* Vered Benhorin, "Music, Psychology, and Motherhood," Baby in Tune, http://babyintune.com/about/.

160   *The visit got me thinking about a movie:* The Music Never Stopped, http://www.imdb.com/title/tt1613062/.

160   *an actual patient as described by neurologist and writer:* Oliver Sacks, "The Last Hippie" in *An Anthropologist on Mars: Seven Paradoxical Tales* (New York: Vintage Books, 1995).

162   *An innovative theater program in Lenox, Massachusetts:* Bessel Van der Kolk, *The Body Keeps Score: Brain, Mind, and Body in the Healing of Trauma* (New York: Viking, 2014), 342.

162   *Van der Kolk describes how the director Kevin Coleman:* Ibid., 344.

162   *Van der Kolk quotes Tina Packer:* Ibid., 345.

163   *In the afterword of his book:* M. Gerard Fromm, ed., *A Spirit That Impels: Play, Creativity, and Psychoanalysis* (London: Karnac Books, 2014), 250.

Chapter 9: Listening for Loss: Time and Space for Mourning

165   *In his book* The Examined Life: Stephen Grosz, *The Examined Life: How We Lose Ourselves and Find Ourselves* (New York: W. W. Norton & Company, 2013), 114.

171   *a beautiful, if exquisitely painful, expression:* Hanya Yanagihara, A *Little Life* (New York: Doubleday, 2015), 163.

173   *A lovely and important blog:* Catherine Keating, "To the Fed Ex Man Who Judged My Parenting Skills," *Pregnancy After Loss Support: Choosing Hope Over Fear While Nurturing Grief* (blog), June 1, 2015, http://www.pregnancyafter losssupport.com/to-the-fed-ex-man-who-judged-my-parenting-skills/.

174   *A recent study in Denmark:* Bjørn Bay, Erik Lykke Mortensen, Dorte Hvidt-jørn, and Ulrik Schiøler Kesmodel, "Fertility Treatment and Risk of Child-hood and Adolescent Mental Disorders: Register Based Cohort Study," *The British Medical Journal* (July 5, 2013): 347.

176   *An op-ed in the* New York Times: Patrick O'Malley, "Getting Grief Right," *New York Times*, January 10, 2015.

180   *A Riggs publication:* Austen Riggs Center, A *Patient's Perspective*, September 2014.

180   *French psychoanalysts:* Françoise Davoine and Jean-Max Gaudillière, *History Beyond Trauma: Whereof One Cannot Speak Thereof One Cannot Stay Silent* (New York: Other Press, 2004).

181   *Singer-songwriter Dar Williams:* Dar Williams, "After All live in concert Te-aneck, New Joisey," YouTube, March 14, 2009, https://www.youtube.com /watch?v=Z0m-4t-Wx9Q.

182   *In one paper, "Speaking Silence,":* Robyn Fivush, "Speaking Silence: The So-cial Construction of Silence in Autobiographical and Cultural Narratives," *Memory* 18, no. 2 (2010): 96.
          S. J. Brison, *Aftermath: Violence and the Remaking of a Self* (Princeton, NJ: Princeton University Press, 2002), 51.

182   *Research by Fivush and Marshall Duke:* Robyn Fivush, Jennifer G. Bohanek, and Marshall Duke, "The Intergenerational Self Subjective: Perspective and Family History," in *Self Continuity: Individual and Collective Perspectives*, ed. F. Sani (New York: Psychology Press, 2008).

182   *described in a* New York Times *article:* Bruce Feiler, "The Family Stories That Bind Us," *New York Times*, March 15, 2013.

184   *through a program bringing unaccompanied children:* "One Thousand Children," Wikipedia, https://en.wikipedia.org/wiki/One_Thousand_Children.

Chapter 10: Listening with Courage: The Value of Uncertainty

188   *In her highly acclaimed collection of essays:* Leslie Jamison, *The Empathy Exams* (Minneapolis, MN: Graywolf Press, 2014), 5.

189   *"As soon as the mother and infant are separate:* D. W. Winnicott, "The Theory of the Parent-Infant Relationship," in *The Maturational Process and the Facil-itating Environment* (New York: International Universities Press, 1965), 50.

189   *In a paper entitled "On Curiosity":* Edward Shapiro, "On Curiosity: Intrapsy-chic and Interpersonal Boundary Formation in Family Life," *International Journal of Family Psychiatry* 3, no. 1 (1982): 74.

190   *Winnicott's view includes a belief:* D. W. Winnicott, *Playing and Reality* (Lon-don and New York: Routledge Classics, 2005), 88.

191   *While Winnicott recognized the value of classification:* D. W. Winnicott, "Clas-sification: Is There a Psychoanalytic Contribution to Psychiatric Classifica-

tion?" in *The Maturational Process and the Facilitating Environment* (New York: International Universities Press, 1965), 139.

191   *"Just like the digital codes of replicating life:* Ian McEwan, *Saturday* (New York: Anchor Books, 2006), 262.

192   *Psychologist Gary Marcus:* Gary Marcus. "The Trouble with Brain Science," *New York Times*, July 11, 2014.

192   *Shortly before the* DSM 5 *was published:* Thomas Insel, "Transforming Diagnosis," National Institute of Mental Health (blog), April 29, 2013, http://www .nimh.nih.gov/about/director/2013/transforming-diagnosis.shtml.

192   *The NIMH is in the process of developing:* "Research Domain Criteria (RDoC)," National Institute of Mental Health, http://www.nimh.nih.gov/research -priorities/rdoc/index.shtml.

193   *In an article about psychiatric medication use:* Thomas Insel, "Are Children Overmedicated?" NIMH (blog), June 6, 2014, http://www.nimh.nih.gov /about/director/2014/are-children-overmedicated.shtml.

193   *Recent research reveals that biological explanations:* G. Schomerus et al., "Evolution of Public Attitudes About Mental Illness: A Systematic Review and Meta-analysis," *Acta Psychiatrica Scandinavica* 125, no. 6 (June 2012): 440–52.

193   *A 2014 study from the department of psychology:* M. S. Lebowitz and W. Ahn, "Effects of Biological Explanations for Mental Disorders on Clinicians' Empathy," *Proceedings of the National Academy of Sciences* (October 2014).

193   *In his tome on depression:* Andrew Solomon, *The Noonday Demon* (New York: Scribner, 2001), 22.

194   *A recent study showed that at age six:* A. Belden et al., "Anterior Insula Volume and Guilt: Neurobehavioral Markers of Recurrence After Early Childhood Major Depressive Disorder," *JAMA Psychiatry* 72, no. 1 (2015): 40–48.

198   *In his paper "On Curiosity," Shapiro uses the term:* Edward Shapiro, "On Curiosity: Intrapsychic and Interpersonal Boundary Formation in Family Life," *International Journal of Family Psychiatry* 3, no. 1 (1982): 69.

200   *National Institutes of Health–funded researchers:* "Common Genetic Factors Found in 5 Mental Disorders," NIH Research Matters National Institutes of Health, March 18, 2013, http://www.nih.gov/researchmatters/march2013 /03182013mental.htm.

203   *In a study of over 300,000 children:* Walid F. Gellad et al., "Geographic Variation in Receipt of Psychotherapy in Children Receiving Attention Deficit/ Hyperactivity Disorder Medication," *JAMA Pediatrics* 168, no. 11 (November 2014): 1074–76.

203   *Another study reviewed over 1,500 charts:* J. N. Epstein, K. J. Kelleher, R. Baum, W. B. Brinkman, J. Peugh, W. Gardner, P. Lichtenstein, and J. Langberg, "Variability in ADHD Care in Community-Based Pediatrics," *Pediatrics* 134, no. 6 (December 2014): 1136–43.

204   *Research has demonstrated that an individual:* M. Nikolas et al., "Gene × Environment Interactions for ADHD: Synergistic Effect of 5HTTLPR Genotype and Youth Appraisals of Inter-parental Conflict," *Behavioral and Brain Functions* 6 (2010): 23.

205   *I wrote a blog post about:* Claudia M. Gold, "The Autism Label Controversy: A Child's View," *Child in Mind* (blog), January 22, 2012, http://claudiam goldmd.blogspot.com/2012/01/autism-label-controversy-childs-view.html.

205   *An irate reader, Landon Bryce:* Landon Bryce, "Pediatrician Claims to Speak for Autistic Children About Diagnostic Changes," *thAutcast* (blog), January 23, 2012, http://thautcast.com/drupal5/content/pediatrician-claims-speak -autistic-children-about-diagnostic-changes.

205   *In the wake of the recent CDC:* "CDC Estimates 1 in 68 Children Has Been Identified with Autism Spectrum Disorder," Centers for Disease Control and Prevention, March 27, 2014, http://www.cdc.gov/media/releases/2014/p0327 -autism-spectrum-disorder.html.

206   *Andrew Solomon beautifully articulates:* Andrew Solomon, *Far from the Tree: Parents, Children, and the Search for Identity* (New York: Scribner, 2012), 222–94.

206   *We see this very problem in Steve Silberman's:* Steve Silberman, *NeuroTribes: The Legacy of Autism and the Future of Neurodiversity* (New York: Avery, an imprint of Penguin Random House, 2015).

206   *In her review of the book, Jennifer Senior writes:* Jennifer Senior, "NeuroTribes, by Steve Silberman," *New York Times Sunday Book Review*, August 17, 2015.

207   *Winnicott's musings on the subject:* D. W. Winnicott, "Autism," in *Thinking About Children*, eds. R. Shephard, J. Johns, and H. T. Robinson (New York: Da Capo Press 1996), 198.

210   *A graduate student at Massachusetts Institute of Technology:* Phech Colatat, "A New Look at Autism's Rise," MIT Sloan School of Management, June 6, 2014, https://mitsloan.mit.edu/newsroom/2014-autism-spectrum.php.

214   *At long-term follow-up study:* William J. Barbaresi et al., "Mortality, ADHD, and Psychosocial Adversity in Adults with Childhood ADHD: A Prospective Study," *Pediatrics* 131, no. 4 (April 2013).

215   *I came across a beautiful expression:* Simon Critchley, "The Dangers of Certainty: A Lesson from Auschwitz," *New York Times*, February 12, 2014.

216   *"I meant what I said and I said what I meant:* Dr. Seuss, *Horton Hatches the Egg* (New York: Random House, 1950).

Index

About the Author

Claudia M. Gold, MD, is a pediatrician and writer with a long-standing interest in addressing children's mental health needs in a preventive model. She has practiced general and behavioral pediatrics for over twenty-five years, and currently specializes in early childhood mental health. She is on the faculty of William James College, University of Massachusetts-Boston Infant-Parent Mental Health program, the Brazelton Institute, the Berkshire Psychoanalytic Institute, and the Austen Riggs Center. She is the author of *Keeping Your Child in Mind: Overcoming Defiance, Tantrums, and Other Everyday Behavior Problems by Seeing the World Through Your Child's Eyes*, and writes regularly for *Psychology Today* and for her blog *Child in Mind*.

Dr. Gold lives in Egremont, Massachusetts, with her husband and children.